The Nature and Treatment of Stammering

First published in 1931, *The Nature and Treatment of Stammering* looks at the theories and causes of stammering as they were understood at the time. It looks at the various treatments available, exposing those 'quack' remedies that are unlikely to work and may make things worse. Then goes on to describe new treatments with proven successful outcomes. Today it can be read in its historical context.

I0095343

The Nature and Treatment of Stammering

E. J. Boome and M. A. Richardson

Routledge
Taylor & Francis Group
LONDON AND NEW YORK

First published in 1931
by Methuen & Co. Ltd

This edition first published in 2025 by Routledge
4 Park Square, Milton Park, Abingdon, Oxon, OX14 4RN

and by Routledge
605 Third Avenue, New York, NY 10017

Routledge is an imprint of the Taylor & Francis Group, an informa business

Publisher's Note
The publisher has gone to great lengths to ensure the quality of this reprint but points
out that some imperfections in the original copies may be apparent.

Disclaimer
The publisher has made every effort to trace copyright holders and welcomes
correspondence from those they have been unable to contact.

A Library of Congress record exists under LCCN: 32002338

ISBN: 978-1-032-93431-0 (hbk)
ISBN: 978-1-003-56588-8 (ebk)
ISBN: 978-1-032-93440-2 (pbk)

Book DOI 10.4324/9781003565888

THE
NATURE AND TREATMENT
OF STAMMERING

BY

E. J. BOOME, M.B., Ch.B., D.P.H., T.D.

DIVISIONAL MEDICAL OFFICER, LONDON COUNTY COUNCIL

AND

M. A. RICHARDSON

SENIOR ASSISTANT, L.C.C. REMEDIAL COURSES FOR STAMMERING CHILDREN

Aequam memento rebus in arduis
Servare mentem
        —HORACE, *Odes*, II, 3, 1

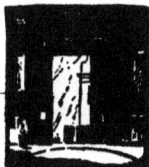

METHUEN & CO. LTD.
36 ESSEX STREET W.C.
LONDON

First Published in 1931

PRINTED IN GREAT BRITAIN

PREFACE

THE authors wish to express their grateful thanks to those who have helped and encouraged them in this work, particularly to C. B. Coxswell, Esq., Dr. James Kerr, Professor John Macmurray, and Dr. C. J. Thomas.

E. J. B.
M. A. R.

LONDON
April 1931

CONTENTS

CONTENTS

THE NATURE
AND TREATMENT OF
STAMMERING

CHAPTER I

INTRODUCTORY

IN the early part of 1927, at the request of the
Board of Education, an investigation was made
into the results obtained by the methods of
treatment in the London County Council Centres
for Stammering Children. Forty-nine unselected
cases were investigated by the medical officers in
charge of the centres, which had all been discharged
one year or more previously as cured or much
improved. The results were to be judged after a
personal interview with the child, together with
any information obtainable from the school and
the parents.

The classification was very strict ; and of the
forty-nine, twenty-four were found to be cured,
nineteen much improved but with occasional difficulty, five improved but still having relapses, and
one worse. In the nineteen much-improved cases
the slight hesitancy shown did not appear to be
different in character and degree from that shown
by non-stammering children of a nervous type.

They were, in fact, regarded by parents and teachers alike as cured. Many more than the forty-nine were seen, but could not be included, since the conditions laid down were not complied with ; that is to say, the child was interviewed, perhaps, but not the parent, or vice versa. The results of these, however, would have been consistent with the figures mentioned above.

In one case the home, when visited, proved to be a barber's shop, and when the patient's father was asked for, a smart youth answered and went in search of him. The father, on learning the reason for the visit, said, ' You have just been speaking to the lad,' and added that his son never stammered now. The boy was one of several assistants, and his colleagues were very much interested to hear that he used to stammer, and immediately did all they could to make him do so for their amusement. The boy, however, returned gibe for gibe with the utmost fluency, and completely foiled their repeated attempts to upset him.

At another home the mother expressed her delight at her boy's cure, and said that, on looking back, she thought the responsibility of the stammer lay with herself. She had always been a very rapid talker, and had often been unduly impatient with the boy's slower efforts at speech. The lad in question is now doing well as assistant to his father, who is a builder.

The fact that, among all the cases investigated, there was not one out of employment, indicates fairly conclusively that stammerers are by no means socially inefficient. The investigation also proves that those cases which resist treatment are the victims of environment, and emphasizes the importance of what may be called the social treatment. The more that is known of the home conditions and of the type of parent, the better the chance of dealing successfully with the patient.

One wishes that the medical profession as a whole would take a greater interest in the important subject of stammering and its treatment ; it has for the most part been ignored by general practitioner and specialist alike. Too often the only advice given by a medical man to the anxious parents of a stammering child is that nothing can be done for him, and that the disability will probably be outgrown. One must deplore such misplaced optimism, founded upon the fact that a certain small number of stammerers do 'grow out of it'. Mason says : 'A boy will grow into it but not out of it', and much valuable time is often wasted because the patient is 'still quite young' and 'there is plenty of time '.

'With the responsibility of human suffering on one side, and the intricacies of the human organism on the other side, who has greater need of a logical mind than the physician ? Who meets more problems in a day—problems as difficult of solution as they are wearing on the nerves ? Who has more general problems thrust upon him with impelling urgency—carcinoma, poliomyelitis, and all the rest ? Shall he sacrifice the credit he has won for the solution of many such problems, and the credit he expects for the solution of the others, by illogical work in this side field, which, though large in the aggregate, is comparatively insignificant. To do so would be to confess lack of logic.' So says Tompkins ; and Mason reports that ' Many years ago . . . a controversy ensued, the result of which was to prove that the treatment of speech defects, by those who have made them their special study, no more intrudes upon the province of the medical man than do the services of the drill sergeant in the school. The one teaches to walk well and the other to talk well. This principle is now universally acknowledged, and acted upon by the great body of the medical profession.'

We are, unhappily, forced to the conclusion that ' the great body of the medical profession ' still holds to this opinion, with the result that the treatment of stammerers has, for many years, been mainly in the hands of quacks and charlatans. These extort large sums of money from their unfortunate clients, and, too often, have only some trick or mannerism to offer as a cure—a substitute which is in general even more embarrassing to the sufferer than the stammer itself. To quote Mabel Oswald : ' Such methods of treatment obviously could not cure, and have done much harm in making the general public distrustful as to the possibility of a genuine cure.' Wyss, also, says : ' The majority of the methods of treatment that enjoy a certain popularity, thanks to clever advertisement, mostly result in a temporary cure only. . . . Among these so-called cures, the stammer recurs after a time with its former severity.'

Again, many are treated by the well-meant efforts of those skilled only in phonetics, voice-production, elocution, etc. In other words, the cure is attempted on speech-training lines, and the important psychological factors are either ignored or treated as of less than secondary value. Ball bears this out when he says : ' The instruction given and treatment prescribed by many so-called professional curers of stammering, instead of relieving, actually *confirm and aggravate the difficulty*, rendering it frequently almost incurable.' And to refer again to Tompkins : ' . . . It is the universal custom to teach stammering under the guise of curing it. But why was not the discovery made before now that the exercises were injurious ? There are three main reasons. The stammerer showed improvement during the treatment, and his temporary improvement was published as a cure, but his relapse was not published.'

Faulty treatment may be partly the result of classification. Stammering is *still* listed among ' speech defects ', whereas it should be under some such heading as ' nervous disorders '. Gillespie, for instance, classes it among ' Habit Disorders ', with which he includes nail-biting, thumb-sucking, incontinence, constipation, vomiting, etc.

Lisping, lalling, and distorted articulation, these are speech defects, among which stammering should never have been included. Had a more correct classification obtained, who knows but that many might have escaped adding to their original trouble the sense of failure and disappointment due to treatment on wrong principles.

Much is being done for the physically defective or crippled child, but very little for the child who is disabled in speech ; and for the stammerer least of all. It is often forgotten that this child lives in a world of his own which is frequently one of prolonged martyrdom. In fact, the child lives in a little hell which is not of his own making : the victim, often, of his parents, his teachers, and sometimes of his doctor.

CHAPTER II

THEORIES

WHAT is stammering ? The *Oxford Diction-ary* says that to stammer is ' To falter or stumble in one's speech, especially to make one or more involuntary repetitions of a consonant or vowel before being able to pass from it to the following sound '. Stammering is equivalent to the German ' *stottern* ', the French ' *begayer* ', and the ' stuttering ' of some of the American writers. In this country ' stuttering ' is no longer used, as it led to confusion ; ' stammering ' covers all forms of the disorder.

Formerly, authorities tried to differentiate between stuttering and stammering by saying, for example, that stuttering was a physical and stammering a psychological defect ; that stuttering was a rapid repetition of any one sound (c-c-c-cat) and stammering an inability to produce voice ; that stuttering was a halt on consonants and stammering a halt on vowels ; or, again, that stuttering was a disorder met with only in young children which developed into stammering if incorrectly treated. Such confusion in terminology arises probably by the differences between one stammerer and another, which appear to demand some such form of classification. But since it may be said that no two patients exhibit a precisely similar stammer, each individual's particular form, on this basis, would strictly require a label of its own.

Many authorities are now agreed on the inadvisability of differentiating between the terms, and we prefer to adhere to the word stammering as representative of all forms of the disorder.

The multiplicity of theories, archaic and otherwise, which have arisen from time to time, show that, in the past, little was known of the origin and causation of stammering. The subject appears invariably to have been approached from every angle but the right one. We do not propose to take an historical survey of these theories. The ground has been covered most adequately and comprehensively by Alfred Appelt amongst others, to whose books the reader may be referred for any information concerning the gradual growth of insight into the subject.

We would, however, make a passing reference to one or two theories which have been advanced from time to time ; and we feel that Burton's ingenuous hypothesis should, on no account, be omitted. In 1660, in *The Anatomy of Melancholy*, he wrote that 'standing waters, thick and ill coloured, such as come forth of pools and moats . . . cause foul distemperatures in the body and mind of man . . . and Bodine supposeth the stuttering of some families in Aquitania, about Labden, to proceed from the same cause'. This is no more absurd than the theory formulated more than two hundred years later that stammering is entirely due to a contest between speaking and swallowing. The author is at great pains to explain in detail—unfortunately not altogether anatomically correct—that the muscles used in swallowing are identically those employed in speech. He contends that, in the former operation, these muscles draw backwards ; while in the latter they work in a forward direction. Accordingly, it is the contest set up by the swallowing movements which impedes speech and makes the stammer. The remedy suggested is delightfully simple : when about to speak the sufferer should not swallow.

The opinion that defective breathing is the cause, and not the effect, of stammering, is still held by many writers of the present day, and by a very large majority of the lay public. McCormac is, therefore, hardly to be blamed for announcing in 1828 his ' discovery ' that the cause of stammering ' arises from the patient endeavouring to utter words, or any other manifestation of voice, when the air in the lungs is exhausted, and they are in a state of collapse, or nearly so. In this consists the discovery, hitherto made by none ; or if made, not announced. . . . I began my investigation with the supposition, that stammering was in general a vicious habit of speech, whose origin and real nature remained yet to be discovered. I commenced with calling to mind the mode of utterance attempted by stammerers ; and I repeated to myself, with all the correctness with which my imagination was capable, the procedure which stammerers employ when speaking or about to speak. By the practice and consideration of these means, it suddenly occurred to me, that stuttering was such as I have already informed the reader, an attempt to speak when the lungs are in a state of collapse. But still it seemed so wonderfully simple, that although I could trace no fallacy in my deductions, I resolved not to be satisfied until I had put them to the test of experiment.'

According to Bluemel, 'the stammerer's difficulty is transient auditory amnesia; he is unable to recall the sound image of the vowel that he wishes to enunciate'. Or, as Paccini puts it, ' Primarily stammering results from transient amnesia which temporarily inhibits the arousal of the necessary antecedent verbal image, of whatever type—visile, audile, or mobile.' Tompkins condemns this theory as fallacious, and we agree with him. If a stammerer fears difficulty with any given word, he resorts wherever possible to a synonym. How could he do this if he had lost the sound image of the vowel, and how could one of normal hearing constantly suffer from such an amnesia ? It would presuppose deafness, or at least defective hearing, in most stammerers. Actually, however, defective hearing and stammering are rarely found in combination. In 522 cases at our Centres we found only 4 with subnormal hearing; Makuen found only 3 per cent in 1,000 stammerers, and in these cases he considered the deafness to be in no way related to the disability of speech.

We find it equally difficult to accept the view that stammering is an aphasia. In the first place, aphasia is usually attributed to some organic disturbance in the brain, whereas a stammerer is, as a rule, perfectly sound organically. Again, aphasia is a partial or complete loss of speech, while stammering is a loss of control or co-ordination of the speech

apparatus ; it is, moreover, spasmodic and intermittent, and in these respects, too, differs from
aphasia.

Tompkins' theory of ' speech interference ' is one
which we find applicable to many of our cases, and
according to him, it accounts for the origin of
stammering by imitation and association. 'The
imitator fears he may "catch" the disorder, he
makes a conscious speech effort in order to avoid
catching it, and by that very effort he makes it
catch.' Thus, any illness, shock, or fright may
cause the patient to make misdirected efforts,
resulting in interrupted speech, which, by drawing
his attention to the mechanism of articulation,
induces further consciousness of what should be an
automatic action.

Of late years the works of Freud and his followers
have attracted much attention, and have been
widely used and abused. Freud's contention that all
neuroses are due to infantile sexual fixations has
aroused considerable controversy. So much has
been written by Freud himself, and so much more
by his disciples, on this subject that we do not
consider it necessary, in a work of this kind, to deal
exhaustively, or in detail, with his theory.

There would seem to be two trends of thought in
the present day as to the causation of stammering.
The one attributes the disturbance to some infantile
repression of an erotic nature ; the other seeks it
in the child's environment. Of the first school
Coriat is an outstanding example, and his work has
been widely discussed. According to his thesis, not
only is the stammer itself the result of some infantile

sexual fixation, but every manifestation of the condition is evidence of such eroticism. He states, for instance, that 'the oral libido in stammering is, therefore, a regression to or an unconscious residue from the pregenital phase of development'. And 'so persistent are the lip-sucking movements in some stammerers, so strong are the movements of the tongue in attempts to speak, that Abraham's term of " Oral masturbation " may well be applied to these manifestations'. Not only do we find it difficult to follow such reasoning, but it is not borne out by our experience in the treatment of children. The fact that a few isolated cases may be traced to a sexual cause does not confirm its universality. Is it not possible that the mistake of viewing the child from the adult standpoint may be responsible for such an outlook ? As Gillespie says : 'One caution must always be observed. It is a caution of interpretation. We must be careful not to play the Lewis Caroll or the Kenneth Grahame, measuring what we observe in a child's mind in terms of adult knowledge and experience. It may seem superfluous to issue such a caution to those who are brought face to face with a similar situation in treating the physical illnesses of children, but in psychological affairs we are far more apt to interpret what we see not merely in terms of adult experience in general, but of our own in particular.'

In our experience Knight Dunlop's theory would also apply to a very limited number of cases only. He contends that stammering is due to the early use of profane or obscene expressions ; that 'the boy who has no great fear or scruple about letting out his gutter vocabulary . . . never . . . becomes a stammerer, but the boy who is carefully brought up . . . a stammerer of the deadlock type. He is always fearful of letting out some obscenity ! . . . It is the proper little boys who become stammerers.' On the other hand, we have had at our Centres many a boy of the type that ' has no great fear of letting out his gutter vocabulary ', and who is yet a stammerer, often one of the most severe cases.

That stammering is a nervous disorder, and not a mere speech defect, is gradually being recognized, although the complete sequence of mental processes is, as yet, inadequately known. As Millais Culpin says : ' Intuition has been in advance of medicine ; the actor or the story-teller will employ a stammer to represent terror or embarrassment, thus demonstrating that its emotional significance is understood.' Munsterberg is of the opinion that ' Abnormal fear is also the essential factor in most cases of stammering. The patients usually know themselves.' And according to Mabel Oswald, ' it has now been established that stammering is dependent on a psychic cause with which it is necessary to deal adequately. Hence the original cause of the speech defect is psychical, the stammer being the expression of a memory of some painful nature which is either wholly or partially repressed.'

CHAPTER III

CAUSATION—I

THE etiology, or causation, of stammering may be considered under two headings :

Endogenous or constitutional, by which is understood a neuropathic tendency with an hereditary proneness to stammering, or an inborn liability to nervous disturbance due to instability of the nervous system. Congenital and physical defects may also be included as Primary causes.

Exogenous or environmental factors, such as shock, fright, illness, or strain, are usually the Secondary or Determining elements. It must be clearly understood, however, that these are never, in themselves, the origin of a stammer. They are occurrences which, by weakening the patient's powers of physical and psychical resistance, discover the latent tendency, that is to say, the Primary cause.

We wish to emphasize the vital importance of investigating the causal factors, if the treatment is to meet with any measure of lasting success ; and we propose therefore to consider these Primary and Secondary causes in considerable detail.

Heredity—' Most men are believers in heredity until the son makes a fool of himself ', said Lord Dewar ; the controversy of heredity versus environment remains unsettled.

Derhardt attributes 78 per cent cases of stammering to heredity; Makuen found 39 per cent with relatives who stammered; on the other hand, Forshaw asserts positively that imitation and not heredity is the essential factor. McMinn says: ' I am not disposed to believe much in the hereditary transmission of stammering, as I have known several instances where the children of inveterate stammerers have never had the slightest trace of it.' The fact that, in these ' several instances ', the children were fortunate enough to escape inheriting the parents' neuropathic condition is hardly sufficient evidence upon which to refute the doctrine that such a characteristic is frequently inherited. We might have drawn the same conclusion from the case of a woman of thirty who had stammered from the age of thirteen, following an attack of chorea. Her three children showed no signs of stammering in spite of the constant example, but we would hardly be justified in looking upon this as sufficient proof that the disability is not inherited. McMinn continues: ' On the other hand, if a child inherits its parent's timorous nature it is bound to stammer from imitation of the parent.' What, then, of those cases in which the parent ceased to stammer before the birth of the child ? Imitation can hardly be said to account for the condition.

' The history is often given of stuttering of a distant relative, seen rarely or never by the child ', says Caroline Osborne, and this statement is borne out by one of Wyss' cases : ' In the G. family . . . there were two stammering children. But the first died of fever before the second was born. The parents, and other members of the family living in the neighbourhood, did not stammer, but a paternal uncle and a maternal aunt, who did not live in the same village, and whom the children had never seen, suffered from this defect of speech to a moderate degree.'

Among 522 of our cases we found 179 with stammering ' in the family ', but we incline to the view that the child inherits peculiar neuropathic tendencies which predispose him to stammering, rather than the view that the actual stammer is inherited.

Pre-Natal Influences must often have an effect upon the nervous system of a child, and many cases have come to our notice where neuropathic symptoms appear to be directly traceable to excessive worry or anxiety upon the part of the mother during pregnancy : anxiety, for example, because of the absence of the father on war service, or his unemployment. In one case, where the stammerer was the youngest of a large family, the mother heard, six weeks before his birth, that her eldest boy was reported wounded and missing ; three months later she heard that he had been killed. Another mother said that her husband knocked her about brutally during pregnancy : of the twins born, one died at birth ; the other, a highly nervous child, stammered. Another father was neurasthenic, and subject to fits, of which he had several just before our patient was born.

One mother witnessed the Silvertown explosion just before the child's birth, to say nothing of air-raids immediately before and after. She had the added anxiety of a husband in the war zone. Another mother had been alone so much during pregnancy that she became permanently nervous. She lived, at that time, in an isolated cottage after having been used to town life, and her husband was obliged to be away for days together. The child began to stammer when, at the age of three, he had to attend hospital for 'starved nerves'. He was a highly-strung child, sensitive, excitable, terrified of noise, and afraid of the dark.

In two separate cases the mothers attributed the speech-disturbance to the fact that they had associated with stammerers in the months prior to the birth of the children ; in both cases the children in question were the only stammerers in their respective families. Another mother said that, two months before our patient's birth, a neighbour 'turned on her' suddenly and abused her loudly for several minutes. The mother was rendered momentarily speechless by the attack, and when it was over she wanted to cry, but found herself unable to do more than 'shudder inwardly'. Her boy, she said, did the same thing when hurt or emotionally upset, instead of crying.

Post-Natal Influences—'Careless handling of the child in the early hours of life may give and fix a habit of fear which is the cause of incipient nervousness and the forerunner of all kinds of neuro-muscular instability', says Caroline Osborne.

We have had several cases of children born during air-raids, and a considerable number where a raid in the days immediately following the birth of the child, causing an attack of nervous hysteria in the mother, appears to have reacted deleteriously

2

on the infant's nervous system. A similar case is that of a child born abroad and brought to England at the age of six weeks, who was rendered so ill by the roughness of the voyage that his life was seriously endangered. Again, one mother was very ill with influenza when her son was born during a bad air-raid; he at once caught the infection. Another mother was unconscious for a fortnight after giving birth to triplets, two of whom died. The surviving boy, our patient, was extremely irresponsible and erratic, unsatisfactory in work and conduct at school, and thoroughly unstable generally.

Rheumatism.—Investigation of a number of cases points to rheumatic fever, or sub-acute rheumatism, as a factor in the causation of stammering, the common association of which with chorea, that greatest cause of inco-ordination in children, is well established. So closely is the latter related to stammering that cases of chorea have been sent to us as stammerers. But in all cases the fact underlying the muscular inco-ordination is the nervous instability so often symptomatic of rheumatic disorders.

Rickets, too, has a much greater effect on a child's mental condition than is generally realized; it leads to a state of general instability of the nervous system, and, in extreme cases, such symptoms as head-nodding, convulsions, etc., may result. In fact, any condition of debility, causing a badly-nourished brain and nervous system, may lead to an irritable condition of the nerve centres and to a consequent lack of muscular co-ordination generally, often affecting the speech mechanism. This condition is so marked in some of our stammerers that it is found necessary, after an initial course in one of our treatment Centres, to send them away for a complete change of air and environment.

The following is a typical case of extreme nervous instability as a result of rickets : Florence Z., a girl of eleven, was born during the war, and her condition was said to be due to under-nourishment owing to the lack of fats obtainable for both mother and child. She received treatment for the rickets, all traces of which disappeared ; but the nervous instability remained, possibly augmented by the fact that both her parents were left-handed, although they had been taught to use the right hand. Florence was a highly-strung child, very excitable, and talked in her sleep ; her speech was excessively rapid, as were her movements, and she had all the restlessness and lack of concentration and repose that are typical of such a child. Her stammer was continuous, though it was never bad enough to interfere seriously, so far as could be noticed, with work or play. She made very little progress, and after a time refused to concentrate. Finally, treatment had to be postponed until she was prepared to make definite efforts on her own behalf to overcome the instability that effectually prevented any improvement.

Left-Handedness.—The connexion between left-handedness and stammering has, in our opinion, been overstressed ; many, nevertheless, still regard stammering as a natural consequence of left-handedness, and maintain that the two are frequently coincident. There are, of course, instances of left-handed children developing a stammer through being forced to use the right hand, but in our experience they are rare; and since schools are increasingly allowing left-handed children to follow their bent, the connexion with stammering is likely to become yet more rare. When these cases occur it is probably lack of confidence, resentment against authority, or the sense of strain consequent upon using the less expert hand that determines the same cause, and may easily develop the inferiority complex which appears to be almost inseparable from stammering. This last may be enhanced, too, by the ridicule which so many people accord to the left-handed.

Investigation into the incidence of left-handedness among normally speaking children in two separate elementary schools, compared with our stammering cases, gave the following results:

Among 280 non-stammerers, in the one, 24 were left-handed, or 8·57 per cent.

Among 350 non-stammerers, in the other, 26 were left-handed, or 7·44 per cent.

But

Among 522 stammerers, 23 were left-handed, or 4·4 per cent.

According to these figures the number of left-handed children among normal speakers would appear to be about double the number found among stammerers. But, although 23 only were left-handed, we found that 132 of the 522 had left-handed relatives, which points to a possible connexion between the left-handed temperament and stammering. The problem, has, however, been extensively treated in Millais Culpin's book *The Nervous Patient*, to which the reader is referred for a detailed analysis of the subject.

Enuresis.—There is no doubt that enuresis—when there is no muscular weakness, mental defect, or parental inadequacy—is a nervous complaint, and one that is often found among stammering children, or in their family history. In one case, for instance, where the family consisted of three children, aged respectively nineteen, seventeen, and fourteen, all began speech with a slight stammer which only the youngest retained, but the other two developed enuresis, from which they still suffered intermittently at the ages mentioned above. The fixation of this habit is often due to the attitude adopted by those in authority over the child and to the unwise suggestion used by them. The child is often accused by his parents of being callous and of refusing to make any effort to improve. He is not callous, but hopeless, and when at the Centre for stammerers he finds that his difficulty is treated with sympathy instead of with blame, he fixes avidly on the simple, common-sense advice given him. Many rid themselves entirely of this habit during the first weeks of attendance at a Centre.

A shock to the nervous system may result in enuresis—one little girl began at the age of six, when her parents had to move from a decent neighbourhood to a very rough district—and occasionally an accident or illness will cause a relapse in a highly-strung child. In cases of enuresis blame is seldom of any use ; but as soon as the child realizes that the remedy lies with himself, he is, in nearly every case, grateful for advice and zealous in carrying it out. Gillespie says : ' Incontinence can also be present as the result of mental conflict, as the non-specific expression of an emotional disturbance, or, more directly, as a self-assertive phenomenon and sometimes as an erotic one.'

Imitation is certainly found to be the determining cause in a considerable number of cases. One boy, for instance, began by imitating a stammering vendor of fish who came periodically along the street ; the boy never missed an opportunity of ridiculing this man, with the result that his condition became yet more marked than that of his model ; and several of our cases have been traced by their mothers to the singing of an erstwhile popular song, ' K-K-K-Katie ' !

Imitation may always be suspected, apart from heredity, when the younger brother or sister of a stammerer follows suit, or when the parent of the child still stammers.

Playing with a stammering child, or sitting next to one in school, is another source of origin in a limited number of cases. It should be clearly understood, however, that association with a stammerer cannot have harmful results, except in one who has a predisposition to stammering ; if this were not so, one would have to segregate those unfortunate enough to suffer from this condition, as they would be a constant menace to their associates. Courtlandt MacMahon bears this out when he says : ' A stammering boy at school is no danger to others unless they are predisposed to stammering.' We are constantly informed that the patient is the only stammerer in his family, or in his class at school. Caroline Osborne, too, says : ' To an observing, imitative child, the speech of another child who stutters may be provocative of trouble. Yet a healthy skepticism [*sic*] as to this being causative as much as it is supposed to be, is aroused by the fact that it is the rule and not the exception to find only one of a family who stutters. If imitation were as baneful as it is said to be, the whole community would long ago have lapsed into hopeless stuttering.'

Defects of Hearing and Vision are seldom in themselves the cause of stammering, but where they exist they are nearly always instrumental in increasing or in fixing the trouble. The unceasing strain to hear or to see involved in ordinary school-work, for instance, makes it impossible to do much for the child's speech until this strain has been removed or at least alleviated.

' Those which be halfe deafe do speak but stutteringly ' (*Oxford Dictionary*, 1615).

The strained and painfully anxious expression of the ' halfe deafe ' child is known to every teacher, and is intensified when the child is also a stammerer ; as has already been emphasized, however, the two defects are seldom coincident.

The number of cases with hitherto undetected errors of refraction is a comparatively large one. Occasionally the provision of glasses appears to be all that is needed to complete the cure of a stammer ; in other cases, where defective vision is one of several complications, a marked improvement is nearly always noticeable as soon as the eyestrain has been removed.

We occasionally number among our cases a few children who obstinately ' forget ' their glasses, or who are incessantly ' having them mended '. This, of course, points to these patients as being more than usually irresponsible, which, combined with the eye-strain, keeps them lingering in a Centre months —nay, years—after they should have been ready for discharge.

Some children suffer from those types of squint that are instances of disorder of co-ordination, and are further evidence of a neuropathic inheritance ; this condition is found even more often among relatives of the stammerer than in the patient himself. In one little girl this squint was extremely marked on her bad days ; it was, in fact, an index to the variations of her nervous condition. It was interesting to watch the eyes gradually adjusting themselves as the child allowed herself to relax in the peaceful atmosphere of the Centre. She arrived many times with the squint distressingly in evidence and would lose it completely after half an hour of relaxation.

Tonsils and Adenoids. — In the past, enlarged tonsils and adenoids were also considered to be a cause, *per se*, of stammering, but this theory is now universally recognized as erroneous. They have no greater effect upon the actual speech of the stammerer than upon that of the normal speaker. It is not the *physical* factor that makes adenoidal children stammer, but the *psychical*. Enlarged tonsils and adenoids fill up the buccal cavity, causing obstruction and a sense of discomfort; when they are removed there is a feeling of uneasiness and a lack of confidence. It is the psychical factor which determines the stammer. In the many cases traced directly to the removal of tonsils and adenoids the cause is usually operation shock or anticipatory fear.

Shock.—In fact shock, mental or physical, may frequently be said to be the determining cause of a stammer, as the following instances show:

Thomas Y., at the age of three, when playing with some older children, was locked into a large, dark stable as a ' joke '; the key was mislaid, and it was a considerable time before the boy was released. Though he had not stammered before, he was now stammering badly.

Albert X. had stammered ever since his father caught him playing with fire and shook him violently.

John W. had scarlet fever at the age of four, and was taken to hospital, where an impatient nurse threatened to ' throw him out of the window if he didn't stop crying '. The stammer had definitely developed when John's mother fetched him away.

Henry T., when he was nine, was pushed off the pier into the water by a rough companion; this not only started the stammer, but set up a species of water-phobia and a terrible fear of the dark.

Mary U. began stammering after the shock of

having several teeth extracted ; the stammer in her case was accompanied by acute jaw spasm.

Walter V. developed a stammer, and a habit spasm that almost amounted to chorea, after a number of operations to his throat.

CHAPTER IV

CAUSATION—II

STAMMERING and Mental Deficiency.—In the past stammering was often looked upon as a sign of mental deficiency. Even to-day many people hold the view that because a child stammers he must be in some way deficient or defective mentally.

The proportion of stammerers among mental defectives appears to be about the same as among children of normal intelligence, but they are much more difficult to cure. In high-grade cases there is generally a psychotic element super-imposed on the original mental defect; these children will be nervous and restless, and lack of concentration and of muscular co-ordination will be more marked and harder to combat than in the normal child.

Raciology.—Stammering would appear to be partly influenced by climate and by the nature and degree of civilization acquired in different countries. It is, for instance, rare in Rumania, Spain, Portugal, and Italy, the lands of soft sounds and of the warm climate which precludes rush and hurry. Again, those countries whose people have fewer repressions and inhibitions, and consequently less mental conflict and nervous strain, will produce proportionately fewer stammerers. In Germany and Poland stammering is very common. ' Indeed,' says James

Kerr, ' the explosive articulatory style of the German school of speech may be contributory.'

Negroid races rarely stammer in their own country; but Dr. Shrubsall, who was in the United States in 1925, says that negroes working among the white population frequently do so. The nervous strain involved in adjustment to civilized conditions, with their complicated actions and reactions, may be mainly responsible for this; to say nothing of the inferiority complex which is such a marked characteristic of the negro living among the white people.

Wallin notes the following ratios between the stammerers of the white and coloured races at Elementary, High, and Special Schools :

	Elem.	High	Special
Coloured. . .	0·6	0·6	} 6·1
White . . .	1·6	1·2	

The head master of a large Jewish School in London, where the racial origin of the pupils is extremely varied, says that the incidence of stammering among Jewish children is almost double its incidence among Christian children ; and Mary K. Scripture and Otto Golgan refer to the speech conflict which is the natural consequence of cosmopolitan cities as a definite etiological factor in stammering.

Age of Onset.—It will be seen from the following table of 477 consecutive cases that there are certain clearly-marked stages in the normal development of every child which, being periods of mental or physical stress, may be in themselves sufficient to account for the onset of stammering, given the pre-disposition. These periods may also temporarily intensify a stammer that is already established.

Years	Boys	Girls	Total
2	83	11	94
3	47	11	58
4	54	12	66
5	63	15	78
6	31	10	41
7	36	13	49
8	32	7	39
9	22	10	32
10	11	1	12
11	5	—	5
12	2	—	2
13	1	—	1
	387	90	477

The first stage is certainly that of learning to talk, when undue attention to childish defects may set up that dread or anxiety which fixes the trouble in so many instances. Further reference will be made to this in a later chapter.

The second stage occurs during the latest period of speech development, the fourth or fifth year, which in the Elementary School is usually coincident with the beginning of school life. The majority of stammerers are very active-minded children, in whose brains ideas are formed more quickly than the power to utter them, co-ordination of the speech mechanism being still imperfectly adjusted. A highly-strung, intelligent child becomes over-excited in his eagerness to express all that is passing through his mind ; his expression shows the strain of his efforts to articulate ; and it must not be forgotten that he is further handicapped by a limited vocabulary and difficulties of selection.

Next comes the period of second dentition, and again we find that the Elementary School child doubles his difficulties by making a change in his school life which his richer brother is spared until at least a year later as a rule. To the nervous child the move up into the big boys' or girls' part of the school can be alarming, added to which the intelligent child often finds himself in a class mostly composed of older children, and the stammer will be the result of his over-eagerness to keep up with the rest of the class.

The attainment of the age of puberty can hardly be said to cause stammering. By the time a child has attained the age of twelve the trouble has usually been established for several years. Very few, however, escape an exacerbation of the defect at this age. In a boy, the change of voice alone is partly responsible for a considerable loss of confidence and increase of self-consciousness during the period of adjustment.

The physiological processes which a child has to undergo at this stage will often affect his whole personality and outlook : he loses confidence in himself ; he tires easily after mental or physical effort ; he feels moody and irritable, ' out of sorts '

generally. Often he resents authority, and becomes
rude and unmannerly ; and he is unable to account
to himself for his ' contrariness '. This can hardly
fail to affect his stammer, and we have seen many
serious relapses with patients between the ages of
twelve and fifteen. Joyce T., for instance, and
Amy S., both attending the same Centre, were so
much affected by the onset of puberty as to be unable
to utter a syllable without terrible effort and spasm.
Both had been progressing favourably before they
suddenly relapsed, and both remained in this almost
speechless condition for nearly a year. Eventually
Amy began slowly to advance, leaving poor Joyce
behind. The improvement continued steadily during the following seven or eight months, when Joyce,
who had apparently made no progress, suddenly
caught up with her friend, and both were discharged,
cured, some weeks later. Again, Jane Q., whose
health was considerably upset at this time, became
impertinent, sulky, and defiant ; she was often
definitely rude and was always difficult to deal with,
until her health improved, and with it her behaviour.

Oliver P. was a case in which a slight delay of
puberty was responsible for a painful relapse into
stammering, whilst its onset produced a rapid cure.
He had been the only boy in his class at school with
an unbroken voice ; for months his inferiority sense
had been increasing, and he had been refusing to
play with his contemporaries, consorting entirely
with those younger than himself. The first ray of
light came when he saw the ' character ' which his
head master gave him on leaving school. Oliver
brought the letter to show us at the Centre, and was

touchingly gratified and surprised to find that his powers were rated so highly, and that his head master had such a good opinion of him. Within a fortnight of this he was visibly 'growing up'; his voice began to deepen, his appearance and carriage to improve, and in less than three months he had lost all trace of his stammer. We found, too, that on Robert O., another case of delayed pubescence, a feeling of uncertainty in regard to his future had been instrumental in preventing progress, and that, as soon as his father, at our suggestion, definitely arranged for him to take up the type of work that he had always wanted, his improvement in outlook, and consequently in speech, was noticeable.

This fear of the future is often a marked feature of adolescence, and particularly so in stammerers, sometimes even remaining with the individual for many years. One patient, for instance, at the age of twenty-one said that he often wished he were back at school again; it was evident that he was wistfully remembering the freedom from responsibility which he had enjoyed while he was living under the definite rules and regulations of school life. This fear of responsibility, and the realization that he will shortly be expected to take his place in the world, will in many cases cause a sudden, last-moment relapse in a child who is about to leave school without having achieved a complete cure. We find, however, that the majority of these cases, as soon as they are settled in their new surroundings, recover rapidly from the temporary set-back and make short work of the little stammer that remains.

CHAPTER V

CAUSATION—III

THE **Difficult Child.**—' The " difficult " child
we know too well; eager, thin, pale,
wasting his little body with the intense
energy which he puts into the whole business of life; a
bad sleeper, a notable refuser of food, often squinting
or stammering, or incontinent of urine, and especially
subject to strange " bouts " or " turns " or
" attacks " as the mother calls them, marked by
increase of pallor, by prostration, by a furred tongue,
foul-smelling breath, constipation, irregular pyrexia,
and so forth.' So says Cameron, and we seldom
examine a dozen children at our Centres without
finding one—sometimes two or three—answering to
this description; and that ' intense energy ' makes
them extremely difficult subjects. They find relaxation almost impossible at first; they make agonizing
efforts to speak; they are incredibly strung up and
anxious, and constantly defeat their own ends by
over-eagerness. One sometimes hardly knows where
to begin with children of this type.

Susan N. was such a child, and one whose life
has been composed of a series of events calculated
to upset the strongest nervous system. She was
born ' blue ', the umbilical cord being wound so
tightly round her neck as nearly to strangle her.
She began to stammer as soon as she started to

speak, and became much worse when, at the age of four, she contracted scarlet fever and was taken to hospital, to which she had to be readmitted with diphtheria three days after her return home. Shortly after this she scalded herself severely. When she was six she had to have two teeth extracted, one of which had formed an abscess ; her mother wanted her to have gas, but the dentist refused, with the result that Susan is terrified of dentists and, up to the age of fourteen, would not allow any one to look inside her mouth. Her house was one of those flooded in 1928, and the violin to which she was devoted was irreparably damaged.

Susan was small for her age, very thin, and painfully nervous ; she talked in her sleep and was terrified of thunderstorms ; she was afraid of fire in any form and would not even strike a match. She was very imaginative and would play ' pretend ' games by herself for hours, a confirmed introvert. She had rheumatic pains, facial tic, and defective vision, in addition to an acute stammer. Susan's progress has been so slow as to be imperceptible for months at a time, but she has latterly improved much more rapidly, and we feel that she is, at last, within a few months of a definite cure.

We find—again with Cameron—that most of these ' difficult ' children benefit greatly by extra sugar ; not only should they have a larger quantity in tea and puddings, but we recommend barley sugar in addition, and with excellent results in nearly every case. Charles L.'s progress, for instance, had been disappointingly slow, and he relapsed badly with the onset of puberty when he started to grow rapidly. Three months of extra sugar had most beneficial results ; speech, energy, appearance, all showing remarkable improvement.

Fear.—Stammerers are never wholly free from fear, although many are so unconscious of the emotion as to deny its existence—fear of breaking down—fear of making fools of themselves, fear of failure or defeat. They often know themselves to be in a vicious circle in which fear and the stammer act and react on each other until there appears to be no way of escape.

Whether or not the patient is conscious of the fear that is causing him to stammer, he gives conclusive proof of its existence in the strained tension of his whole person ; muscular tension being the inevitable result of fear of any kind.

One's first duty towards a stammerer, then, is to help him to relax the mental strain under which he lives ; to tell him that, by practising deliberate muscular relaxation he will gradually acquire greater ease of mind, which will, in its turn, restore self-confidence and self-respect, and will, by degrees, eliminate the fear of speech.

The determining cause of the stammer, in many of our cases, has been traced to the repression of some concrete or imaginary fear or dread, which when brought into the open can be dispelled by discussion. Of late years it has no longer been thought cowardly to admit the presence of fear ; it is now fully recognized that, especially when hidden or repressed, it is a great cause of present-day neuroses. Prolonged worries, anxieties, and fears, however small, take their toll of mental energy, and, sooner or later, unless brought into the open, will react deleteriously upon the mind as a whole. This is usually enhanced in a patient with a neuropathic tendency, and especially in a stammerer, business or family worries causing an intensification of the speech disturbance. Often the mere discussion of what the patient has hitherto repressed will cause an immediate relief, and in the ensuing treatment progress is usually fairly rapid.

Some people may go through life without ever experiencing the emotion of fear, but they are in the minority, although many can say that they have never known the sensations of extreme terror. The effect of a terrifying experience may not be immediate ; a well-known airman is said to have remarked that, although he felt no actual fear at the time of his exploits, it took him seven years to recover from the strain of which he was unconscious at the time. Charles Lamb wrote on this subject : ' I was dreadfully alive to nervous terrors. The night-time, solitude and the dark, were my hell. The sufferings I endured in this nature would justify the expression. I never laid my head on my pillow, I suppose, from the fourth to the seventh or eighth year of my life —so far as memory serves in things so long ago— without an assurance, which realized its own prophecy, of seeing some frightful spectre.' And ' I durst not even in the daylight, once enter the chamber where I slept, without my face turned to the window, where my witch-ridden pillow was. Parents do not know what they do when they leave tender babes alone to go to sleep in the dark. The feeling about for a friendly arm, the hoping for a familiar voice, when they wake screaming, to find none to soothe them, what a terrible shaking it is to their poor nerves.' Or to turn to Burton's description : ' Many lamentable effects this fear causeth in men, as to be red, pale, tremble, sweat, it makes sudden cold and heat to come over all the body, palpitation of the heart, syncope, etc. . . .

' Many men are so amazed and astonished with fear, that they know not where they are, what they say, what they do, and that which is worst, it tortures them many days before with continual affrights and suspicion. It hinders most honourable attempts, and makes their hearts ache, sad, and heavy. They that live in fear are never free, resolute, secure, never merry, but in continual pain.' Nothing could better describe the mental state of a stammerer than those final lines.

The following cases illustrate the impossibility of effecting a permanent cure while fears remain repressed.

Julius M. was seven when he first came to us. The history was very bad—insanity on the father's side and acute nervous instability in the mother's family ; the boy himself was highly nervous and physically debilitated. The stammer had started suddenly about a year previously, but the mother was most emphatic in denying any shock or upset having caused it. Julius was discharged some two years later, apparently cured. He returned to the Centre at the age of twelve and a half, stammering more severely than on the first occasion, after an acute attack of rheumatic fever. It was only then that we learned, during a talk with the boy, that a year before his first admission he had had a serious shock. He and a younger sister were alone together when she set fire to herself ; Julius, then only six, tried frantically to attract their mother's attention, but was unable at once to open the door. His little sister was so badly burned that she died on reaching the hospital. The subject had never since been mentioned at home, and as a result of the nervous disturbance caused by the shock and its suppression Julius had convinced himself that he was to blame for the other child's death. The accident had to be discussed with him several times before he began to lose the sense of guilt, and with it the acute increase of stammer brought on by the first mention of the word ' fire '.

Another case is that of George K., who came to a Centre at the age of twelve. He was in a highly nervous condition and had a marked squint, for which he wore glasses ; he was abnormally afraid of the dark, refusing to sleep except with the light full on and the door open. George had lost his mother when he was five, and his father being away at sea most of the year, he had until twelve months previously lived with an aunt, who had a large family of her own. Since then he had been living with friends of his father's, who were very fond of him and anxious to do their utmost for him. To the best of his foster-mother's knowledge the stammer was first noticed when he was eight years old, at which time he was moved from a small private school to the Elementary School. The foster-mother thought that the boy's aunt had been too strict with him, her own children being robust and free from ' nerves '. George was very shy, and was inclined to shun boys of his own age, feeling more at ease with his juniors. From the boy himself we learnt that when with his aunt he and an older brother shared a room at the top of the house. George had always feared and disliked this brother, who used to tell him ghost stories every night, until he was afraid of going to sleep for fear of dreaming of them. Later, his brother having gone abroad, and George's room being wanted, he was moved downstairs to sleep on a couch in the sitting-room, and found himself the only occupant of the ground-floor at night. His terrors increased, being augmented by the fact that the scullery roof jutted out under the sitting-room window, and he could hear ' cats and things ' walking on it. Then came the move to his foster-mother's house, by which time the very act of going to bed was fraught with fear, because it was always the prelude to terrifying dreams.

He had never before told any one of the reason for his terrors, and the discussion of the situation seemed to bring immediate relief. It was suggested to him that he should practise relaxing in bed at night, as he was learning to do at the Centre, and that he should accompany this with the reiteration of an auto-suggestion formula to replace the ' terrifying thoughts ' of which he complained. The effect of following these instructions was unexpectedly rapid. At the end of a fortnight the boy informed us that he had told his foster-mother she might turn out the light so soon as he was in bed, and that she might shut the door.

In another instance a highly-intelligent little girl of seven owned to an overwhelming fear of rain. We had considerable difficulty in finding the reason for this, but finally she admitted her conviction that whenever it rained it was the beginning of another Flood. The subject had to be discussed on several occasions before the terror vanished. It is probable that many passages in the Old Testament are capable of arousing such terror in the mind of a sensitive, imaginative child, and the same may certainly be said of the stories of bloodshed and disaster which pass sometimes as ' fairy tales '. The robust and healthy child usually glories in such stories ; is he thereby working off a certain amount of superfluous sadism, or is it equally bad for him, although in a different way, as it is for the highly-strung child, in whom such narratives may evoke endless night terrors ? A boy of eleven, for example, had a recurring nightmare about Red Indians after reading a book in which the phrase ' he cut off his head and hung it on his belt ' made such an impression as to haunt his imagination for months. Unfortunately, the more a child broods over a fear of this description, the less likely is he to speak of it, and it is just this repression that is so harmful. Once the matter has been discussed it loses its terrors.

CHAPTER VI

SYMPTOMS

FACIAL Expression.—Nearly all stammerers, unless their affliction is a very mild one, bear a strained and anxious expression, and the more severe cases exhibit, in addition, an appearance of definite sadness and depression, these symptoms being accentuated when the patient attempts to speak. The stammerer is never free from the dread of breaking down ; he not only feels this when in the act of speaking, he is perpetually anticipating and dreading the event, consciously or unconsciously, and his facial expression is therefore a true index to his mental state.

Tension.—A greater or lesser degree of hypertonicity is inseparable from stammering, and in acute cases the whole muscular system is affected. When such a patient is tested his whole body is found to be tense and strung up, his arms and legs are rigid, as are the muscles of the thorax and larynx ; the jaw and tongue are equally tense, and there will probably be very bad laryngeal spasm as soon as he is asked to speak. Respiration is jerky owing to the inhibitory action of the chest muscles, and expiration may be completely held up for as long as five or six seconds. On auscultation at the bases of the lungs there is frequently a suspension or marked diminution of respiratory murmur. The diaphragmatic action is likewise out of order, and the length of time during which expiration is inhibited may be due to sudden diaphragmatic rigidity, no less than to the faulty costal movement with which it may be combined. In such a case a corresponding rigidity will be noticeable in the abdominal muscles, through which control of the diaphragm is to a large extent obtained.

Spasm.—Rigidity and spasmodic movements are, unfortunately, not confined to the actual mechanism of speech, nor are they only in evidence during the process of articulation. In many stammerers the simplest gesture lacks rhythmic co-ordination, and it is often painful to watch their contortions when attempting speech. Some patients, for example, will repeatedly jerk the head backwards or forwards ; others will preface speech with violent movements of the arms or legs ; others, again, will exhibit facial twitchings, eye-blinking, or clenching of the jaw. These spasmodic movements might almost be called a substitution stammer, the muscular spasm continuing until speech is effected, when the stammer proper supervenes.

Excitability.—On the mental side, too, one finds a variety of symptoms, of which a general excitability is usually the first mentioned by the stammerer's parents. In fact, he often ' only stammers when he gets excited ' ; many of this type, however, appear to be in a perpetual state of excitement, and consequently of stammering. They can never take events calmly ; they rush into action or speech, seldom allowing themselves to do either quietly ; and they naturally have no conception of the meaning of repose and relaxation.

If children of this excitable temperament combine with it a constant restlessness and irresponsibility, they become extremely difficult subjects for treatment in a class. The presence of one child of this description may upset the repose and quiet of the others, while his inattentiveness and continual fidgeting may cause serious disturbance, and may definitely retard the progress of the class as a whole. This extreme irresponsibility is, fortunately, not a characteristic of the majority of stammerers, and it is usually confined to the younger children. Even so, however, two such attending simultaneously have been known almost to wreck the work of the remaining ten at a Centre, and their presence in a class constitutes a serious problem for the instructor.

Emotionalism.—Stammerers, in common with other highly-strung individuals, are often very emotional and easily elated or downcast ; they are extremely sensitive to ridicule, and are quickly embarrassed by any signs of tension or impatience in their hearers. Patients of this type are usually morbidly introverted, worrying continuously about their speech difficulty ; they are always on the watch for a relapse, and frequently cause it by their anxiety ; they discount any improvement in their condition by looking upon it as merely temporary, and will often, by their mental attitude, lengthen by many months the time required for a cure. Even when the improvement is so definite that they cannot ignore it, they find some other aspect of the case to worry over ; in fact they bear out Richard Aldington's apt comment in his *Death of a Hero*, that ' " worry " is not " caused " by any event ; it is a state which seizes upon any event to " worry " over.'

Other patients, adults as well as children, may possess that volatile temperament which prevents them from continuing treatment to the end. These will work with great enthusiasm until a certain point is reached beyond which they seem incapable of going ; they then lose interest and either stop short, sometimes within actual sight of the goal, or begin gradually to regress.

Sense of Inferiority.—Adler tells us that, just as most diseases depend upon some constitutional organic anomaly and a physical attempt to compensate for an inferior organ, so in the psychic field an inferior organ may give rise to an unconscious feeling of psychic inferiority and to compensatory mental mechanism. According to this theory, neuroses and psychoses are the results of unsuccessful compensation ; anxiety is an outstanding and common expression of the failure to compensate for some defect ; and stammering is frequently a feature of an anxiety neurosis. Instances of psychic compensation are seen in the assumed self-assertion of the timid : one indulges in over-dressing and vulgar ostentation ; another assumes a loud voice and a boastful manner. Defiance and resentment against authority or a general 'naughtiness' are often symptoms of this same inferiority sense— symptoms in which the victim pretends to glory while inwardly he is miserably aware of failure.

It is often said of stammerers that they push themselves forward ; that they positively seek opportunities for speaking ; and even that they do not mind stammering and never avoid a chance of doing so. If we might only enter the minds of these sufferers for a few hours, and understand what they are really feeling under all this apparent ' bluff ', we should then realize to some small extent the martyrdom which they ceaselessly endure : a martyrdom aggravated by a constant sense of failure in spite of their most gallant efforts. ' They often disguise under an air of indifference and tranquillity, the anguish of their hearts at their miserable infirmity.' So writes Forshaw ; and a young man once poignantly said to us : ' I often feel I would like to go somewhere right away and lose myself.'

Wendell Johnson, in his book *Because I Stutter*, gives a living and moving description of the trials, hopes, and fears of a stammerer. It is one of the few books written from the patient's own point of view, allowing one to see into the inner recesses of his mind, and bringing out clearly the reactions of a stammerer to the world, and the world's attitude to him. The following extract is typical : ' Stuttering is a mental distraction and a physical drain on the energies of the individual. It interferes with his work in school especially, not only because it forces him to think of himself constantly as being something of an exile, but also because the process of stuttering makes him in the moment of stuttering, far less capable of carrying on the thought process than he otherwise would be. . . . Stuttering is a constant mental and physical pain, and although the stutterer learns, in time, to regard this pain nonchalantly, it remains important and can never be wholly disregarded.'

' Defected minds, timorous and tame and low spirits are hardly ever to be raised, and very seldom attain to anything,' said Locke in 1690. This sense of inferiority, although by no means confined to stammerers, is one of the characteristics which they all share in common, and which is largely due—in a child, at any rate—to environment. Constant fault-finding and discouragement can only be withstood by the strongest and most independent characters; the others are gradually worn down until, from doubting their ability to do well in any given direction, they become quite certain of their inability to do so. Pascal said : ' Man is so formed that by dint of being told that he is a fool he believes it, and by dint of telling himself so he makes himself believe it ' ¡ and a child whose manners, appearance, and achievements are the subjects of continual adverse criticism, can hardly fail to develop a sense of inferiority. If those in the patient's immediate environment would realize that awkwardness, clumsiness, gaucherie, and so on are symptoms of nervous strain, and would try to find and remedy the cause, there would be fewer unhappy and maladjusted people in the world. Unfortunately these symptoms are too often treated with ridicule or punishment, which instead of correcting the trouble only serve to increase it.

Cyril J. is an instance of a boy suffering from a sense of inferiority. He was fourteen years old when he came for treatment, and had stammered since he was five. He came from a good home and his parents were anxious to do all they could to help him. He was the eldest of three children, but neither his younger brother nor his little sister showed any signs of speech disturbance. He was highly intelligent and had won a scholarship, on the strength of which he had been, for the past year, a day boy at a public school. His mother said that his stammer had been severe from the first, but that he had become yet worse after an operation for tonsils and adenoids when he was six, and again on going to his new school a year before we saw him. The tendency to stammer was hereditary, his father having stammered as a boy and his mother's sister having had similar trouble with her speech.

The boy himself was highly nervous and very introverted, and had a distressingly marked inferiority complex which affected his manner and movements generally. He was always very quiet, refused to make friends, and had the additional handicap of being ineffective at games. He was also extremely pessimistic as to the possibility of overcoming his stammer, and it was almost impossible to convince him that he was making progress. He always adopted the attitude that the improvement, if any, was negligible.

During the eighteen months of his attendance at the Centre he was working for matriculation, which he eventually passed, and then left us to take up work. He was by this time very much improved and distinctly happier and more hopeful about himself. When he was seen again, some three years later, he was working in a telephone exchange ; he had lost nearly all trace of his stammer, and the difference in his general appearance was remarkable. His carriage was upright, his expression happy and

confident, and his whole bearing was eloquent of
the change in his mental outlook.

Richard H. is another example. He had infantile
paralysis when he was four years old, and had to
wear irons for years, which, according to his father,
gave him a ' Charlie Chaplin ' walk. When he came
to the Centre at the age of fourteen this peculiarity
was hardly noticeable, and his right leg was only
very little shorter than the left ; the right heel was
slightly raised, but he was able to run and play
games with comparative ease ; he said that his leg
only ached after prolonged walking. He was a
highly intelligent boy who had won three scholarships and was working for matriculation. The
stammer, which was in his father's family, was
moderately bad, but the most noticeable feature in
this case was the marked inferiority sense, evident
in every movement. Improvement was obtained
with this boy by discussions of his very creditable
scholastic achievements as compared with those
of other boys at his age, and comparisons of his
present athletic powers with those of the past.
His intelligent appreciation of his own case was,
we think, the chief reason for the rapidity of
his cure.

Another case, and a very difficult one, was that
of a girl who, although only eleven, was full grown
and broad in proportion, and who towered like a
giantess over the other children at the Centre and
in her class at school. She was painfully self-
conscious ; she had outgrown her strength and was
quite apathetic about her speech, and it was almost
impossible to make her take any interest in the work

at the Centre ; her progress was, consequently, so slow as to be almost imperceptible.

Other cases have come to us who, being very small for their respective ages, suffered from an inferiority sense and a self-consciousness that did much to retard progress.

CHAPTER VII

ENVIRONMENT

ONE sometimes wonders which is the more difficult child to deal with at a treatment Centre, A the spoilt and pampered child, or B the neglected one. A's mother fusses over him, does everything for him, and is constantly and tensely anxious for his welfare ; B's mother does nothing to help him, is not interested in his progress, probably only notices his stammer to 'scream' at him about it or to hit him for it. When the treatment depends almost entirely upon the work carried out by the patient himself, both these types are at a loss, the victims of their environment.

Let us deal with A first. He has the advantage of being well fed and well clothed within the limits of the family purse ; he is often the only child, and yet is not allowed to find companionship because objections are raised to his playing with 'those nasty, rude boys' in the street. After a time he himself prefers not to mix with these boys, since he finds himself so much below their level of achievement, whether in games or mischief. The self-distrust which has gradually been growing now becomes intensified, and his only security is his mother, who is always ready to listen to him, to admire him, and to praise his doings. School, as a place where he has to fend for himself, becomes

50

increasingly distasteful to him, and he will probably be kept at home owing to illness much more often than the average child. This is not an accusation of deliberate malingering, the headache or sore throat are quite genuine, but they arise out of the subconscious wish for something that will interfere with going to school.

By this time his sense of inferiority and his stammer are definitely fixed, and it becomes our task at the Centre to try to alleviate both, with little or no help from the patient. His mother has always done everything for him, let her therefore also undertake the work of curing his stammer ; in fact, the child probably does not know how to begin doing things for himself, and months may be spent in showing him. Usually, he is not even allowed to come to the Centre by himself ; his mother brings him every time, although many a younger child comes the same distance unaccompanied. The mother of a boy of twelve and a half always insisted upon bringing him, and when, after he was thirteen, she had to go out to work because the father was ill, Norman had to discontinue treatment. The head master, when appealed to, remonstrated with the mother, in vain, in spite of the boy's earnest wish to attend. This was not the case of an only child ; Norman was the youngest of the family by several years, and was very naturally beginning to resent being treated as a baby. Although his manners had hitherto been quite above the average, his resentment took the form of being rude to his mother and generally surly and unapproachable at home. It was pointed out to his mother that the remedy for all this was to allow him a certain amount of freedom and independence, but nothing would alter her attitude.

Another instance of a spoilt child is that of Charlie M., who was an only child. He was born prematurely, an eight months' baby, and was *very* delicate during his first year. He was born in the north of England, and his mother believed firmly that his ' native air ' was the only one that suited him, that he never stammered when staying there, that London did not agree with him, that the part of London in which they lived suited him least of all, etc., all of which Charlie had heard discussed many times. The child was backward in learning to talk, and the stammer began when he was five, following an attack of scarlet fever. Two years later he developed whooping-cough, during which illness his mother was confined ; the baby caught the malady and died in a few weeks. Charlie retained a very vivid memory of his little sister and constantly talked about her. The boy never had the chance of learning to be independent or self-reliant. He was watched over incessantly and at the slightest sign of indisposition he was put to bed and kept there. It is significant that, while he was away in the country with other boys, the master in charge reported a complete cessation of the stammer, which was again as bad as ever upon his return home.

At the Centre, Charlie was a constant source of unrest, with his continual fidgeting, his walk and movements were awkward, clumsy and self-conscious, and his grimaces and contortions on attempting speech were painful to witness. It was nearly two years before he showed any definite signs of improvement, and then he did so only very slowly. At the end of three and a half years the boy had made a distinct all-round improvement: his speech was decidedly easier, he had lost nearly all the accompanying spasm, and he had learnt to relax to a fair extent.

By this time he was naturally losing interest in the work at the Centre, and he was therefore discharged in the hope that self-treatment would increase self-confidence. Further reports show that the improvement was maintained, but that he is still far from being cured, which is hardly to be wondered at when one realizes how changeable is his background. He is periodically moved from one school to another because he does not receive enough ' individual attention '; his homework is seldom unaided; he receives advice and guidance at every turn. Yet we feel that he has sturdy, useful qualities; it is his home environment that has prevented their development.

Now let us turn to B, the neglected child. He is usually one of a large family whose mother, through lack of means, overcrowding, endless childbearing and -rearing, has become hopeless and fatalistic. B is left mainly to his own devices; there is no order or discipline at home, and it is a hard task for him to conform to these at school. It is not through the efforts of his mother, but through those of his head master, that a place is found for him at a treatment Centre; often this same head master makes special arrangements whereby B may carry out his daily practice at school, knowing too well that no such facilities will be forthcoming at home. Even so, progress is often depressingly slow. B can hardly be blamed for this when all that is said of the matter at home is that he is worse, or, at any rate, no better. Sometimes he is capriciously withdrawn from the Centre on these grounds.

Harold H. is a typical instance of such a case. He was admitted to the Centre at the age of ten ; he was entirely undisciplined and inattentive ; he took no interest whatever in the help that was offered him ; he was continually naughty in the class and he obviously took no advantage of the opportunities his head master gave him for practising at school. The mother refused to take the trouble of coming to see us, and naturally very few particulars could be learnt from the boy, whose stammer was extremely severe. After eighteen months, when signs of a slight improvement were at length apparent, his mother promptly said that he was getting worse and was to cease attending ! His head master intervened on this occasion, and again a year later. In the meantime the boy's speech had gradually improved, in spite of the small amount of care and interest taken by Harold himself. In this, his fourth year at the Centre, he is working moderately well and is making distinct progress ; personality and behaviour have also changed for the better. Whether a child of this description is capable of definitely curing himself is not certain ; we have seen such unexpected results in apparently hopeless cases, however, that we do not despair, even of Harold.

The following instances have been taken at random

from the many cases in which environmental influences were chiefly responsible for the stammer.

Leslie G. was brought to us at the age of eleven by his father, a man of extremely poor physique. Of a family of seven, only three were alive. The mother was highly strung and had a bad squint. Leslie was a seven months' baby and had had to be kept in cotton-wool for the first six months of his life. The stammer began when he was five, as a result of being knocked down by a motor-van and sustaining injuries to his jaw that kept him in hospital for three months. He had a weak chest and said that he often dreamed that 'a train was going over his chest'. At the Centre we found him restless and inattentive, intensely nervous and excitable, completely lacking in concentration and a general disturber of the peace. He was entirely 'shut in' and reserved until the following information—to which his father had made no reference—was supplied by his head master : when Leslie was nine years old he was led astray by an older boy, and with him used to steal buns from a neighbouring coffee-house. The boys were caught by the police and ultimately Leslie's present head master agreed to admit him to his school in order to keep him from the influence of the older boy. When Leslie found that we knew of this episode at the Centre he was induced to talk about it, reluctantly at first and later with an evident sense of relief that amounted to a modified form of reaction. There was, to begin with, no change in the boy's behaviour as a result of these discussions, he continued naughty and inattentive and made not the slightest attempt at practising

or at carrying out instructions ; but his appearance altered, he gradually lost his furtive expression
and the look of strain and unhappiness ; his health
began to improve, aided by the fact that we were able
to send him away for change of air more than once
during his two and a half years at the Centre ; and
at last, very slowly, and then more quickly, his
speech began to improve. By the time he left
school, and in consequence the Centre, he had very
little stammer, he looked one straight in the face,
he had acquired repose and self-control, and, we
hope, the power to prevent himself from being
dragged down again by his environment.

Bernard F. was a boy whose stammer was quite
obviously due to home conditions. He was born
with rickets, his mother died when he was sixteen
months old and his father shortly afterwards married
again a woman who was completely antagonistic to
the boy, as she was to his sister, who was four years
older. When Bernard came to the Centre, particulars were given us by his uncle, his father having
refused to come because he was ' so fed up with
him '. Accusations of lying and of stealing fantastic
sums from the family purse were laid against the
boy ; he was said to have tried to poison the house-
hold by putting lysol in the tea-pot, to consort with
a gang of undesirable boys, and to be unsatisfactory
in every way ; ' a thorough bad lot '. The father
appeared to agree with this account of the boy and
with his wife's treatment of him. The head master's
account, on the other hand, was a totally different
one ; the boy gave no trouble at school and was a
good, intelligent scholar.

Bernard was apathetic when he first came to the Centre ; he knew that his uncle had poured out a long list of his misdeeds, but he brightened visibly when he found that no distinction was being made between him and the other boys in the class. It took very little time to establish friendly relations and to induce the boy to talk about his troubles. He admitted having lied and stolen—both evidently defence reactions—but emphatically denied any attempt at poisoning. He said that whenever anything went wrong at home he was always accused of being the culprit, that anything that had been mislaid was instantly supposed to have been stolen by him, and that no one ever believed a word he said. Bernard's great ambition, he informed us, was to be a sailor, and he was eager for a complete change of environment that he might make a fresh start. He said that he was sure he could be honest with people that believed in him. With the assistance of his head master, Bernard was sent to a training ship after having attended at the Centre for three months. During this time the stammer had almost disappeared under the influence of renewed hope, and we learnt a year later from his head master, whom he had just visited, that he had made good, that he was a changed being, happy and confident, that he bore an excellent character in his new surroundings, and that he had lost all trace of his stammer.

Nora E. was eleven when she came to us, with an hereditary tendency to stammer, several members of her mother's family being afflicted. The mother, who was highly strung although she had never actually stammered, fell off a bus during her pregnancy, and was again severely upset by a Zeppelin raid three days after Nora's birth. The mother developed breast abscesses, in consequence of which the child had acute gastritis, and both spent many weeks in hospital. Nora added to her troubles at this time by having measles and pneumonia. She did not begin to stammer until she was over five, when her teacher is said to have hit her roughly and knocked her off her form ; this same teacher would never allow the child to read aloud because it ' got on her nerves '. By the time Nora was moved up among the big girls, the stammer had become acute. On the other hand, she now began to enjoy school life instead of dreading it, liked all her new teachers, and was devoted to her head mistress, who was ' ever so nice '.

Nora was highly strung, very restless at night, talked and walked in her sleep, was afraid of the dark and was subject to headaches although there was nothing wrong with her sight. She made excellent progress when she first came to the Centre, and then relapsed. We ascertained that her father, a naturally irascible man, whose irritability had increased since he had been out of work, was continually telling the child that her stammer was increasing and that it ' got on his nerves '. The mother was sent for, and promised that she would speak to her husband and would make things easier for Nora. For a time again all went well, but the father had not sufficient patience, and there was a second relapse. The onset of puberty was now adding to Nora's difficulties ; she was having attacks of giddiness and faintness, and was losing interest in her progress under the stress of constant discouragement ; she appeared to have given up all effort. Other home conditions were further complicating matters : the child was under-nourished ; she was also worrying over her eldest brother's treatment of their mother. He, it seemed, was a ne'er-do-well who lived on his parents when out of work, but whenever he found employment invariably left home and made no effort to help the family exchequer.

The mother refused to come and see us again, and we appealed to the school for help. The head mistress went to a great deal of trouble on Nora's behalf ; she made the mother understand that the child *must* have assistance and encouragement at home and wrote us a detailed letter of the circumstances. Thanks to this intervention on the part of her head mistress, conditions became easier for Nora, and her health and spirits improved, with the result that her stammer had practically disappeared by the time she left school.

In the months prior to the birth of James D. his mother was full of anxiety for her eldest son, who was on active service, and who was killed when Jim was a few weeks old. She herself died when the boy was eighteen months. From that date until Jim was nearly eight years old he was a great deal alone, and one can only surmise the fears that loneliness must have wrought in his mind. We were informed that the stammer was not noticed until he was between five and six years old, but we think that it probably began earlier. Shortly before he

was eight, a sister gave up her outside employment
to live at home. She it was who brought Jim to the
Centre when he was eleven ; she said that he was
very nervous and terrified of the dark. From his
head master we learnt that Jim had been a mastur-
bator when he first came to school, but that latterly
this habit had ceased.

At the Centre we found Jim a depressed boy with
a *very* bad stammer ; he was utterly lacking in
co-ordination and was excessively tense. He informed us that he was one of those people who
always had ' unluck ', and it was impossible at
first to make him admit that he was making any
progress. His advance was certainly slow, but it
was apparent. We were forced too to remonstrate
with his father and sister because they were continually telling the boy that he was ' no better ' or
' getting worse ', After many months Jim was, at
last, ready to acknowledge a definite improvement.
He said that the home comments were still adverse,
but that he now ' took no notice of them ' because
he was convinced that he was better. His reports
from school were good, and he was feeling happier
and looking more cheerful and contented. We
feel that it is now only a matter of time before his
cure is affected.

Maud C. was brought to the Centre at the age of
ten—a very attractive little girl, well brought up
and cared for. Her mother was intensely reserved
and little could be learnt from her. We elicited
that Maud had stammered since she was three and
that she was extremely nervous, but the mother
denied having had any shock or upset during

pregnancy or after the child's birth. A few weeks
later, however, we learnt, through the kindness of
the Care Committee, that the father had been severely
wounded at the time Maud was born ; he had had
to have his nose and part of his jaw grafted on, and
he was very sensitive about his disfigurement.
The whole family reacted to this, and Maud was
born and brought up in an atmosphere of extreme
tension.   Had it not been for a neighbour who was
devoted to the child and who frequently invited her
to spend evenings and spare time with her, the
stammer would, in all probability, have been even
worse than it was.   It was very bad when we first
saw her, with a great deal of accompanying spasm ;
she also had a marked squint, which diminished
somewhat as her speech improved. After some
months with us she won a scholarship to a central
school, and at first the change seemed to result in a
relapse.   However, as soon as she was settled in
her new surroundings and happy in her work she
again began to improve.   Progress was slow, since
it was not possible to change her home environment, but latterly it has been more rapid, and we
hope that she will not have to attend the Centre
much longer.

CHAPTER VIII

THE STAMMERER'S POINT OF VIEW

WE feel strongly that no book dealing with the subject of stammering should omit the point of view of the patient himself; after all, he, and he alone, can appreciate in full the mental state associated with his affliction. To this end we have invited comments from a number of patients, asking them to reveal to us their feelings and reactions. The main object of this chapter is, as we told them, that of helping their fellows, by showing other stammerers that they do not suffer alone, and by giving those who come into contact with stammerers some comprehension of what they have to endure.

The reiteration by totally different persons of similar emotions and conflicts should enhance rather than detract from their significance, and should emphasize the need for their recognition in treatment. At the risk, therefore, of what may, at first glance, appear to be unnecessary repetition, we have extracted, but in no wise altered, the following passages from the comments sent to us by patients whose ages range from twelve years upwards:

(1) ' I was indoors when someone frightened me and gave me a shock. I was speechless for the moment and after that I started to stammer. Some

people make a mockery of me, but I take not a bit of notice of them.'

(2) 'Since I started at school, my only drawback has been my stammer. I have always been afraid of asking for explanations of any subject from the teacher. I think that teachers should have this explained to them.'

(3) 'When my parents, or anybody else, send me on an errand, I keep on saying to myself, "I have to say what I have been sent for", and when I come to the shop and try to say what I want it hardly comes out I feel so tense.'

(4) 'When I am in a shop and I stammer I go all red and I can't get my words out, and the people laugh at me, and I write the thing down on a piece of paper, and then I give it to the man. Sometimes when I am in school and I am speaking to my teacher and I stammer, the children laugh at me and my teacher tells them to leave off.'

(5) 'It is best to be quite frank about your stammering. It is no use bottling it up and thinking to yourself continually, "I wonder if they know I stammer yet", and all that kind of thing. After a while it will only make your stammer worse. Laugh at it and let them laugh at it if they want to.

'If you come to a word in your speech that you cannot say, don't try to say it, it only makes you stammer more, but just hesitate for a second or two and think of another word that means the same thing. Don't worry about hesitating; the person whom you are speaking to will not notice it; every one hesitates in their speech now and again—it is only natural.'

(6) ' I think the general attitude of people towards stammering is rather that of poking fun than anything else, except perhaps a few who have had anything to do with a stammerer. This was illustrated not long ago when a satirical revue was being broadcast. The players were discussing things in other plays in a ridiculing way, and one spoke of a certain play in which a man stammers and he said, " There's plenty of fun in that ".

' People may think a stammerer is not trying to improve, yet many cannot believe that he would not stammer if he could speak like they can. It is very tantalizing for him when he sees every one around him speaking in an effortless way which seems so easy and simple and yet which he has been trying all his life to do.

' When he wishes to say something he may be thinking so much whether the words will come out all right, that when he does speak he gets confused and says the wrong thing or the sentence appears in a different manner. The person spoken to may then get an idea that he is abrupt, that he has bad manners, or that he does not know the correct words to say, and so gets an opinion of him different from his true character.

' Stammerers are placed in extremely awkward positions if they have to keep a person waiting before they can speak. I have been in these situations and have felt relieved when the person stopped talking. But once a stammerer has improved he knows the joy of being able to speak anywhere to anybody he likes, and which, after all, is what most people have always been able to do and think nothing of it, and yet the stammerer has been kept from this happiness through no reason of his own.'

(7) ' Few people really appreciate their gift of fluent speech, but from a stammerer's point of view it is a pity to indulge too much in self-pity ; there is generally some one who stammers worse, and every stammerer has blissful moments of freedom in speech.

' I find that I am really better with strangers. Probably I am worst with the people I am most fond of and know the best, and those that are most anxious for me not to stammer.

' A great help, I find, is to listen to the quality of one's voice, instead of the actual words ; to try and attain a pleasing intonation, and if you like acquire certain mannerisms from other people. For instance, I found that I could manage better if I spoke with a Scotch accent, or better still with a drawl. But of course the only lasting and complete source of help is in relaxation, although only a stammerer knows how terribly difficult that is when speaking.

' I have found it a help to think of quiet and deeply calm country scenes that I have visited alone ; for instance a small, still lake surrounded by unblown willows.

' I am generally better with members of the opposite sex, but have not heard if that applies to most stammerers. At the moment I am trying hard not to think of the actual words of a sentence before I say it, and also not to anticipate difficulties in speech, because fear, of course, is more than half the trouble.

5

' I think many a stammerer is discouraged because so often parents and others will *not* listen to what children say, especially those who are members of a large family. For those who come in contact with stammerers, and there are many, do not look the other way when he or she is in difficulties, and even if it is a great friend never tell him to be quiet however nicely it is said. However much a stammerer laughs at himself, he is extremely sensitive, but I must say that, so far, I have always found the public extraordinarily kind and sympathetic.'

(8) ' I feel that others should realize what a burden stammering is on one's mind. Having stammered all my life until a few months ago, I was sort of inured to it. However, on going to school and mixing more with folk, I was so nervous and shy that I hated speaking to anybody, and I thought that being sent shopping was the worst form of torture. There was one shop in particular where the assistants openly laughed at me. Once I got so exasperated that I flared and gave the assistant a long speech on his facial and other drawbacks. This was accomplished without any stammer ; but unfortunately, when I wanted to speak after that I forced my words as badly as before. However, on being cured I did not mind going shopping ; in fact, I went whenever possible. No longer when I speak to a stranger do I expect him to snigger or burst out laughing as before.

' I very rarely got asked out to tea or to parties because I never spoke a word, and when spoken to only grunted or else made a fool of myself. And even now I have a reputation and have only been to

one party in the last three years. But since moving
to a fresh address I have met new people, and
although I never was good at making conversation
I have never failed to fill up gaps or keep up a flow
of chat in a conversation. This not only makes
me feel bucked with life but gets me asked out
to tea.

' Not having to worry any more about my speech
enables me to work with much more freedom of
thought at school, and all my nerves have gone.
Indeed, I am now in the shooting eight at school,
where nerves and shaky hands are *verboten*. Also,
as a result of the relaxing, my health has improved
both mentally and physically. There is no more
premature tiredness.

' I never had been ragged at school, probably
because I was rather free with my fists, but now the
chaps who occasionally twitted me remark on how
changed my speech is ; and I use my tongue to
scathe them with, whereas before a free fight
generally ensued.'

(9) ' There seems to be little doubt that child
stammerers are very inclined to use their impediment
as a protection. They may find that they are
treated with more consideration at school or at
home, being excused oral questioning, the delivery
of verbal messages, etc. Personally, I am convinced
that this point is of the utmost importance, since
it is not until the necessity for earning one's living
arises that one really appreciates the great drawbacks stammering entails. What is the use of
trying to assist a child who sees no reason why it
should be assisted ? In my case, at least, no

earnest desire to be cured existed until near the completion of my higher school education. I had not appreciated the great disadvantage that threatened my future.

' Regarding my attitude to other people : I had a most strong desire to punch people who attempted to help me out ; such a person immediately gets me into difficulties. Such persons have an uncanny gift of suggesting entirely the reverse of what one intends to say, and, instead of relieving the sufferer, only serve to entirely blot out any self-control he may have possessed. The person who clearly expressed pity was also of great danger to my type of stammering.

' Taken generally my speech was reasonably sound when I met people for the first time—more particularly when they were persons of consequence. Frequently, mental fear or awe of a person really caused an improvement in my speech, rather than the reverse—at any rate, for a short period.

' In my short experience I have found that stammerers in general are very prone to flights of imagination, in which they picture themselves as masters of rhetoric. By thus dwelling on what is far from possible at the time they are quite likely to wipe out any good that auto-suggestion may be doing them. It simply causes a deep despondency.

' I found no more difficulty in speaking foreign languages than in speaking English. French, German, Spanish, and Welsh presented no more trouble in so far as the individual words are concerned than the English equivalent. Even now I get good and bad periods. The good periods are very good

and even the bad periods are comparatively good
to what they were even a short while ago. In
spite of many attempts to discover a cause for
these periods, I have so far failed to reach a satisfactory solution.

' In my type of stammering the reason seems to be
a kind of nervous tension. Undoubtedly the chief
cure is relaxation, but it is a deuce of a job to keep
relaxed.'

(10) ' In perusing these notes, please remember
that I cannot remember NOT STAMMERING. As far
as I, personally, know, I have *always* stammered.

' I *know* I am a stammerer, and when I commence
to talk I am out to say it as well as I can. I talk
differently—well and badly—to different types of
people. Some look at me with annoyance written
on their faces and think they are being hurt at having
to listen to me, and I get the impression that it is
a relief to them when I am gone. This has a bad
effect on me. Sometimes I say to myself bitter
thoughts about the person who has made me feel so
badly my impediment. Other times I forget about
the person, and only a desperate longing to talk
comes over me. To some people I *always* talk badly.
Somehow, their very presence upsets me. They are
not necessarily people for whom I have a dislike,
but their critical look and stare upset me, that's all
I can put it down to. Of course the opposite type
of people I get on very well with. Some are very
sympathetic and *don't help me out of it* ! Which
is just what I want. Other sympathetic hearers do
so (out of kindness, of course), and this makes me
worse, because, if what they say isn't what I intended

saying, I have to say " No ", stop and start again. I think you will see what I mean.

' Sometimes I despair of ever talking well, and in calmer moments realize my folly in letting it get me down. I am really very unhappy about it all. Often in despair (black despair sometimes), I have cried out in my inmost soul that I was never meant to talk—that I was intended always to stammer. But stammering must be fought, and gradually I am learning to take defeats in a good and helpful (to myself) spirit.

' With regard to strangers I vary. When I commence the converstaion, which I do sometimes to get into the way of speaking well, I usually get on fairly well. But when I suddenly hear a voice ask me something, most times I fall and stammer. I could never stand up before an audience and speak, although I could sing without the slightest difficulty. When I was at school I stammered much worse than I do now, and the master used to make me stand out in front of the class and say what I had to say. To me it was a source of intense mortification and chagrin, and it never did me the slightest benefit. The other boys laughed when the master imitated my contortions, and I longed for the end of the school hour when I could go out of that horrid class-room into some quiet spot, alone.'

(11) ' In my own case I have found stammering a great handicap in nearly every department of life. It is very true that stammerers do easily develop an " inferiority complex ", and that it is always more or less apparent : the fear that one may stammer and so become a nuisance to other people.

This occurs often in the following cases : (1) Waiting in a queue for railway tickets or in a shop when there are other customers to be served. (2) When telephoning and giving the number required to the exchange, who *may* be irritable and say two or three times " Number, please." (3) Saying grace at a meal when every one is waiting either to start or to leave the table. (4) When a boy or girl at school and questions are being asked round the class, etc., etc. In all these cases the stammerer, while waiting, gets more and more anxious about how he will speak when his turn comes and whether he will hold up the queue. Whereas, if he goes to the booking-office or into a shop with no one behind him waiting he will at once feel calmer and be able to say what he wants easier.

' In my own case I feel that all the facial muscles are locked and that no sound will come forth because of this spasm. A stammerer has his ups and downs, and I find myself very discouraged when the " downs " come. If I begin a day badly, it generally means that I shall stammer a great deal all day, and by the evening feel quite exhausted with the efforts I have made to speak. The more one stammers the worse the day seems to be and the fear becomes greater. I also find difficulty when asked a question suddenly, even to answer " Yes " or " No " ; but the worst difficulty comes when a question is asked which has only *one* answer ; for instance, the name of a town or a person's name. Immediately the feeling comes I know I can't say it, and there is no way round, no convenient bridge, and the more effort I make to say the name the less result. I have always had tremendous difficulty in saying my own name, whether in a shop, on the telephone, or in private conversation ; that has become a perfect nightmare to me, and I often wish I could change my name, although I am sure the changed name would be just as difficult. I feel I shall stammer when asked my name, so I always try to dodge it, and yet the fear always remains.

' Then, again, when in a crowd of people, in a bus, a train, a theatre, etc., I often have the feeling that every one is looking at me and thinking that I have a stammer. Thus does the stammerer rather belittle himself in other people's eyes ; he tells himself all this hallucination is nonsense, and yet the fear remains and he wishes to hide himself. No one who is not a stammerer can really gauge the true feelings of despair which sometimes come through a stammerer's mind—almost the feeling that he is a hindrance to other people and that he causes others much pain and annoyance.

' I have passed through such times myself, and the main reason must be that the stammerer has lost confidence in himself, that he lives in a constant state of tension, and that he is constantly feeling " worked up " and " on wires " when there is no need to feel that at all. Then it is that the locking motion takes place, and he feels himself incapable of saying anything.

' In my own case I definitely pass through various kinds of stammer in turn : a shivering of the jaw, opening the mouth wide and no sound coming forth, a continuation of the sound " er ", grinding of the teeth, etc. All of these occur in turn, but when the muscles and brain are perfectly relaxed none of these occur.

'I hope very soon to be able to say that all the feelings I have attempted to describe above will be things of the past and merely how I used to feel *when* I stammered.'

(12) 'In the first place I will give my history as regards my stammering. I have been stammering for as long as I can remember, except for a few very early recollections.

'The rather vague border-line between this part of my life and that which followed it is marked by a dream which even now is extremely vivid. I was lying in bed one night facing the wall, when it gradually became transparent and illuminated by a pale green light. Then a clutching hand, dark green in colour, came slowly out of the wall towards me and caught me by the throat. I was too petrified by far to cry out or even move. Then it gradually faded away as it had come.

'From this period the attitude of mind which characterizes a stammerer began to assert itself. I became retiring in disposition and began to be easily depressed by even the most trivial occurrences. During these early years domestic troubles arose which, unfortunately, I was better able to comprehend than most children are.

'It has continued to the present, sometimes only manifesting itself in a little hesitation or stumbling over a difficult word ; sometimes being so severe as to render me absolutely dumb. I have endeavoured to find some relation between stammering and physical and nervous conditions, but I can find no reliable guide. Sometimes I have been better in speech when my physical health has been decidedly below average. During times of nervous strain and debility speech is undoubtedly worse, but when my nerves are in good condition there is not the improvement that might be expected.

'Attitude of mind undoubtedly does play a large part in a stammerer's condition. It is not so much what you expect to do that matters ; it is what you feel like. I have gone up to a person to say something, fully expecting, from previous experiences, to be able to start speaking perfectly easily, and found myself absolutely unable to utter a word. If, on the other hand, circumstances and my frame of mind allow me to regard that person as being inferior, I can assume a patronizing or condescending manner, and most of my difficulty vanishes like magic. The cause of this seems to be fear of criticism.

'Fear of criticism is with me almost a phobia. Almost unconsciously I follow the majority just to avoid being criticized. I say very little, mainly to avoid criticism. I cannot be natural ; I cannot give expression to my ideas, sentiments, and longings ; I have to smother myself in a maddening blanket of restraint. Because I dread criticism I dare not be original ; what would other people think ? Of course it would be unthinkable, monstrous, for me to criticize other people or to attempt to smash *their* cherished opinions. 'The impertinence of him !' And when the inevitable question ' Why ? ' comes, the most that I can do is to stand, red in the face, on one leg, and make curious noises, while some look on in amusement, some in pity, and the person I am attempting in my feeble way to criticize curses impatiently and turns away in disgust to talk to someone else ; every one else drifts away, leaving me hanging in mid-air, as it were, exasperated almost to tears with everybody and everything, especially myself.

' Perhaps I have given some idea of the mental tortures a stammerer has to go through occasionally. Usually I am philosophic about it. I just take it for granted. By means of various ingenious plans I can usually lead a more or less normal, though somewhat restricted, social life. I have stock words and phrases covering a good many of the expressions in general use which I find fairly easy to say, and I use them whenever possible. When a difficult word comes along I can usually, at the expense of grammar or meaning, get round it by using an easier word. But occasionally—especially if my speech happens to be bad one day and I've had to admit that it's beaten me hands down—I give myself over to an intense introspective depression, leading inevitably to the fatal question—Is it worth while ?

' I will now endeavour to give an impression of what stammering feels like to the stammerer himself. I will take a typical incident which happened to me a few days ago. I wanted a morning off to attend a hospital for dental treatment, and as application had to be made to the inspector I knocked and entered his office. He is sitting at his table writing, and looks up inquiringly as I walk in. He knows that I stammer, so I am not afraid of making a fool of myself. I only have a certain feeling of sympathy for him, for I know that it is just as painful for him as for me. He looks at me for a few moments while I compose myself, and then looks down again and starts scribbling on his blotting pad. I know exactly what I am going to say beforehand, so I take a deep breath and force the first word out, after a struggle. But perhaps I am a little premature. The normal person cannot understand a word having to be forced out, so I will try to explain. Take a deep breath and make as if you were going to cough. When you feel your throat contracted in readiness to open again for the expulsion of air under pressure from the lungs in the form of a cough stop short, keeping the throat contracted and the lungs trying to force the air out. You will find that the harder you try to make a sound the more difficult it becomes. If you continue you will become purple in the face and it will feel as though a blood-vessel is going to burst. These are more or less the physical feelings of a stammerer.

' To continue with our little episode : I force the first word out. Now I find all my breath is gone, and if I go on in the same way I shall have the same difficulty with the second word, and so on. Now I discover that my fists are clenched, my whole body is taut, and I am standing on my toes, or even on one leg. Dear me ! I must relax ; I can never speak like this. So I relax, take a deep breath, and, as nothing occurs to divert my attention, I can get enough impetus to carry me through the sentence. When it is all over and I am out of the office again I feel quite exhausted, both physically and mentally, and, coupled with this, that sense of incompetence which many people feel after their best efforts have been defeated.

' I can sing, mimic, and speak alone without the slightest trace of a stammer. If I speak without thinking too I experience no difficulty. But if I have to think before I speak, or if I go into a shop knowing beforehand what to ask for, I have to struggle like mad to get anything out.

' I can usually speak all right to strangers, if the remarks are quite commonplace or unnecessary, such as observations on the weather, etc., but if, as I have just mentioned, I have to ask for something in a shop, or if some one inquires the way off me, the stammer crops up.

' With my friends I am a little better as regards speech, but, even so, I have had some very hard struggles to get a word out, even with my most intimate acquaintances. Among the fellows at work I am all right if I can speak jocularly, but if I have to speak seriously I stammer badly. With those at home I still stammer, but it does not involve the same amount of effort as is usually required to speak.'

While in the process of collecting the foregoing comments, we discovered Wendell Johnson's enlightening book, *Because I Stutter*, and we have extracted the following passages, which, as will be seen, tend to confirm the statements of our patients :

' In more severe instances of stuttering, I have become aware of an increased rate of heartbeat, heightened blood pressure, flushing, perspiration, and trembling. The mental accompaniments have been chiefly dread, anguish, and a longing to escape, to vanish from the sight of those about me. I have felt weak, pathetically mortified, and incapable of speaking. At times I have responded to the restraint which stuttering imposes upon me, by general rage, with its physiological symptoms and its so-called mental flurry and decreased consciousness or awareness.

' This fear of stuttering consists chiefly in the anticipation of difficulty, and it arises from the fact that stuttering has been known to occur before. It does not cause stuttering ; rather it is caused by stuttering that has occurred in the past.

' One attribute is common to all my stuttering : tenseness of the somatic musculatures, more noticeable in the abdomen and shoulders. This is true regardless of the fact that particular sounds are characterized by particular types of stuttering. In the abdominal region this tensity is concentrated because of the restricted contraction of the nearby diaphragm ; in the shoulders it is a function of the prolonged distension or deflation of the lungs and the consequent effect on the attendant musculatures. The effort involved in speaking with difficulty, however, is accompanied by a complete somatic contraction.'

CHAPTER IX

TREATMENT—I

IN an earlier chapter reference was made to a few of the many existing theories that have been brought forward to account for the causation of stammering. What now of the numerous methods of treatment? For while here lies the patient's best hope, here also is real danger. Although a certain number may be honest enough to admit ignorance of the cause of stammering, most people think themselves competent to give the sufferer advice, and nearly always of the 'trick' variety.

The victim is told to tap with his foot, hand or finger; to clench his teeth or his fists. It is true that such tricks will often have a momentarily good effect, by diverting the patient's attention from the speech mechanism, but it is seldom that they do not ultimately increase the stammerer's muscular tension and add to his self-consciousness a sense of failure and depression.

The unhappy victims of these quack 'remedies' will, by consulting books written by 'experts' on the subject, find methods yet more difficult to obey. One system, for instance, insists that the jaw must be kept clenched, not only during speech, but during the preceding inspiration, and that on

no account must the teeth be separated until the
sentence is finished. Upon reference to another
authority, the stammerer learns that he must make
a sweeping downward movement of the lower
jaw for *every* sound, vowel, or consonant. Again,
he is told to raise his head slowly all the time he is
speaking, the head-raising to continue to the end of
the sentence. And so this type of treatment goes
on *ad infinitum*. It would be ludicrous were the
consequences not so serious. Unfortunately, the
stammerer, far from being cured by such methods,
is often made worse. We seldom encounter a
patient who has not been given some form of
' trick ' advice, and the majority of such patients
report an increase of stammering as a result.

One of the worst examples was that of a boy of
sixteen, George B. He was told by his head master
to tap with his hand against his side in time with
the syllables uttered. Up to that time his stammer
had certainly been severe, but when he had made a
habit of the ' tapping ', and it was then that we
saw him, he was literally speechless. He had
derived benefit for the first few days, during which
he followed his master's instructions, and then finding
that he was not being so successful, he had tapped
harder, with the result that tension had become
more severe, and both this and the trick movement
had increased. By the time we interviewed George
he was no longer tapping his side with his hand—
he was hitting it with his clenched fist, and often
jerking his leg as well. His whole body was rigid
with an effort that forced tears to his eyes, and after
minutes of agonizing attempts he would still find

himself unable to articulate. The boy's mental state might be said to be as tense as his physical condition ; he must have had intelligence of a high order to matriculate with credit, as he did, under such a strain.

It was months before George was able to relax when silent, and still longer before he could retain any sense of ease when trying to speak. Needless to say, there was no improvement in the speech until the spasm, and the tension causing it, had given way. And this martyrdom—we can call it nothing less—was the ultimate result of apparently an innocent-looking hand movement. We are thankful to say that his gallant struggle in the face of apparent failure has had its reward. May we hope this account of George's sufferings will spare other stammerers a similar fate ?

Speech Training.—One hears *ad nauseam* of methods based on the need for re-education of speech. Stammerers are required to practise for hours at a time vowels, consonants, syllables, words, and finally phrases. Long passages of poetry and prose have to be memorized, test sentences repeated, and so forth, the teacher ignoring the obvious fact that a stammerer is already obsessed with the mechanism of speech, and that he needs to be led *away* from, and not *towards*, his obsession. To quote Tompkins : ' Normal speech is automatic. Through an accident or incident an individual makes a conscious effort and blocks his normal speech. The resulting conflict attracts ridicule. In order to avoid repetition of the ridicule further effort is made and further impediment results. . . . So - called cures — the

6

breathing exercises, articulatory exercises, and so on—are distractions, and therefore cause an improvement which is represented to be a cure. The trouble with them is that they inculcate conscious speech and thereby intensify the stammering.' Liebman also says : ' According to my view the stammerer makes the mistake of directing his attention too intensively to his speech. Through this basic fault he becomes sensitive to each slight physical interruption, becomes anxious regarding special sounds, and begins therefore to interrupt the progress of his speech by all kinds of unfortunate voluntary speech and breathing efforts.'

The views of a visitor from the United States are interesting when considered in this connexion. Having watched a group of our children going through their breathing exercises, she informed us that at the clinic in which she worked all such exercises were barred since they tended to make the children more self-conscious ; that they were given instead articulatory exercises for which they used mirrors, that they might study the formation of the sounds, the position of their lips and tongues, and so on. None of which was apparently supposed to induce self-consciousness !

It is true that speech training, re-education of speech, elocution—whatever it may be called—frequently results in temporary improvement ; but complete cessation of the stammer is seldom achieved ; so soon as certain limits are reached retrogression usually begins, the stammerer often finding himself worse after ' treatment ' than before he started. In one case the patient told us of having had what he called 'explosive treatment' at the age of thirteen, he had had to practise long lists of words beginning with whatever letters he found most difficult. This method very effectively fixed the obsession, and where the initial letters specified had been difficult they now became well nigh impossible. Many years later he came to us and, referring to his previous experience, he stated that 'B' was one of his worst initials, and that he frequently went without butter on his roll (a successful evasion of the word 'bread') rather than make himself conspicuous by struggling to ask for it.

The stammerer himself should refute the theory that he is in need of speech-training exercises. It is a recognized fact that stammering—unless the affliction be very severe—is intermittent, and during his periods of normal speech the patient supplies proof of the efficiency of his articulatory apparatus. His speech will usually be at its best when he is taken off his guard, and therefore 'thinks aloud' instead of consciously going through the act of speaking. Hence he rarely stammers when alone or when talking to his peers. The absence of difficulty in such circumstances is further evidence against the need for articulatory exercises. Here the greater part of the attention is paid to proper vocalization or voice-production, whilst the enunciation becomes almost subconscious, and effort is therefore eliminated. With some stammerers recitation is on the same level as singing ; especially among Jewish boys, whose dramatic instinct, once aroused, will sometimes carry them unhesitatingly through a long speech. One boy of thirteen, for instance—a very severe case—who had been attending a Centre for about six months, gained a special prize for recitation, although his conversational speech was still far from being cured.

Voice Production. — In studying the various methods advocated for the cure of stammering, it will be found that the majority insist upon what is called proper vocalization, or voice-production, the exponent of each method having his own interpretation of these terms. Most would appear to call upon the stammerer to assume some artificial voice or manner of speech to cover or to take the place of his own faulty production. Often a definitely sing-song voice is required of the patient, or else he is told to make conscious efforts to lower the pitch or to talk in a monotone. Many stammerers are too self-conscious to face the world with this type of voice, preferring the stammer as less likely to focus attention upon them.

The originators of these methods appear to have overlooked the fact that the neurosis causing the stammer is also causing the muscular hypertonicity which results in an unnatural voice, and that once this tension has been conquered, the patient is usually found to have quite a good voice of his own. Why not, therefore, help him to resume his own voice, instead of forcing upon him an alternative that is wholly foreign to him ? The number of stammerers requiring actual exercises in voice-production is no greater than the number of normal speakers in need of such exercises. Even for those with the husky voice previously referred to, ' voice-production ', as understood by the elocutionist, will seldom be found necessary. This huskiness is nearly always due to laryngeal spasm and chest tension, as part of the general hypertonicity. Once the patient has learnt to relax, the tension disappears and the voice becomes normal and natural.

Breathing.—Reference has already been made to McCormac's 'discovery' that stammering was due to faulty breathing. In view of the costal and diaphragmatic spasm present in nearly all cases, it is perhaps not altogether surprising to find that this fallacy still flourishes. To the superficial observer the spasm is sufficient proof that faulty breathing is the cause of the defect, and it is on this assumption that the curative methods of many 'specialists' are based. The general public, and a number of present-day text-books, accept the diagnosis without question, and, filled with good intentions towards the stammerer, instruct him to breathe deeply every time he wishes to speak. The well-meaning giver of such advice can never have tested for himself the effects of 'taking a deep breath' every few words ; we would suggest that he try carrying out his own instructions before advising his victim. He will very soon realize what a laborious undertaking he has recommended to one who is already heavily burdened.

This fallacious theory in regard to a stammerer's breathing is probably based on the prevalent assumption that he does not breathe before speaking. This applies to a few, certainly, but the majority inspire in readiness for speech, and then, owing to rigidity and muscular spasm, are unable to expire, or find that they have not sufficient control to expire evenly.

This inhibited expiration is wrongly accepted as evidence that the stammerer has tried to speak without first breathing. The small amount of breath needed for the short phrases of conversational speech is inspired unconsciously by the majority of stammerers, as it is by normal speakers.

These observations should not be taken as implying that breathing and breath-control exercises are unimportant. When based on principles of relaxation and rhythmic co-ordination they are invaluable as means of inducing confidence and mental ease. Tompkins and others would dispense with them altogether, but we do not think such a course necessary or advisable, especially when dealing with children ; breathing exercises only become harmful if they are made a conscious adjunct to speech. By the time a patient has learnt to relax his muscles, and to *allow* his breathing mechanism to work of itself, instead of *forcing* it to do so, he has relegated it to its rightful sphere, that of automatic action.

Hypnotism, as a cure for stammering, is a subject upon which authorities hold conflicting opinions. Wyllie considers it to have failed so completely as to put its advocates out of court ; Tompkins' view is that it undoubtedly affords relief, but that its permanent effect is questionable ; Wyss, although he advocates hypnotic treatment, allows that retrogression occurs in about 50 per cent of the cases treated, nor does he look upon it as a substitute for ' rational treatment '. ' Hypnotic suggestion and psychoanalysis are the two principal methods of reducing psychic tension, and so eliminating attentive instability,' says Crichton Miller ; while Munsterberg is of opinion that ' every hypnotist can quickly secure a strong improvement—then the improvement becomes slower, and finally it stops before a complete cure is reached. The patient notices it and it easily works back on his emotion, and this begins again to disturb the speech, unless a very careful continuous contrasuggestion is given.'

We feel very strongly that this last statement is only too true, and that it points to hypnotism as a positive danger to stammerers. In our experience we have not found it to be of any permanent value ; it obscures the psychical injury instead of removing it ; and when the artificial control ceases the stammer recurs, rather worse than before ; this happened frequently in war cases.

Why hypnotism when suggestion will suffice ?

CHAPTER X

TREATMENT—II

INVESTIGATION **of History.**—It is of comparatively little use to undertake the treatment
of a stammerer, whether child or adult,
individually or in a group, without ascertain-
ing as much as possible of the family history,
and of the health, mental and physical, of the
patient.

A thorough physical examination should precede
treatment and any defects, such as errors of refraction or enlarged tonsils and adenoids, likely to
retard progress, must be remedied. It is essential,
too, that the treatment be carried out under the
direction of a medical man. When the patient is a
child it is necessary to interview one of the parents,
or some one who stands *in loco parentis*, in order
to elicit particulars of the history and, when
needful, to suggest alterations in régime or in the
general family attitude towards the sufferer. Details
of the child's health and nervous condition, his
general behaviour and characteristics, etc., should
be ascertained.

The importance of co-operation with the Centre
on the part of home and school cannot be too strongly
emphasized. As Dr. W. Allen Daly, when Medical
Officer of Health for Blackburn, in 1924 said : 'The
conclusion I have drawn is that even the worst

cases of stammering are curable when there is co-operation between parent and teacher, and, considering the seriousness of the affliction, at comparatively small cost. In Blackburn cases where there has been complete failure to make progresss in reading, recitation, or conversation, it was owing to the indifference of the stammerer, coupled with the parents' lack of appreciation of the value of the instruction given.'

We are in direct touch, too, with the schools from which are drawn the children who attend our Centres. An invitation to watch a group at work is sent to the teacher of every child three weeks or so after his admission, and, further, the instructor has a definite time set apart for visiting these schools in rotation. Here, as in the preliminary interview with the parent, much valuable information may be obtained as to the patient's outlook and his adaptability to the community, to say nothing of the attitude of schoolmasters in general towards their stammering pupils.

Having learned as much as possible of the stammerer's environment, discussions with the patient himself follow. It is now recognized that the Word Association Test is invaluable as a method of approach to such discussions and to the mental state of the stammerer. It helps to bring to light those conflicts and repressions that are causing the anxiety neurosis, and it gives, too, some indication of the educational level of the child patient.

The test consists in giving a series of stimulus words to which the subject is told to respond with another word as rapidly as possible. Stammerers are, of course, not so quick in responding as are normal speakers, and this must be taken into account when dealing with such patients. The practice, which one occasionally sees advocated, of allowing the stammerer to write his responses, is one that can be productive of little result. If the patient is sufficiently at rest to make the Word Association Test of real value, he will be unable to go through the repeated action of writing, nor do we feel that the response, when written, can be properly spontaneous. Accurate timing, too, must be difficult if this procedure is adopted. We never make use of this test with a stammering patient until he has proved himself at ease in his surroundings, and on confidential terms with the practitioner. Given these conditions, and allowance being made for a modicum of stammering, it may be successfully carried through.

There are various indications whereby it is possible for one experienced in this procedure to determine when one of the stimulus words strikes a buried complex. The most common of these is a PROLONGED REACTION TIME ; either the patient upon hearing the word thinks of a word which he does not wish to say, or else his mind becomes blank, and it may be many seconds before a response is forthcoming. Sometimes this mental inhibition is so strong that there is NO RESPONSE at all, even after a long wait ; the patient will say that he ' can't think of anything '.

Among further complex indicators are ; a REPETITION OF THE STIMULUS WORD, or a pretended MISUNDERSTANDING of it ; the NAMING OF SOME

OBJECT IN THE ROOM, or an emotional reaction such as LAUGHTER, TEARS, or an increase of STAMMERING. All these are signs of an unconscious desire on the part of the patient to evade response.

That, briefly, is the method employed in the Word Association Test ; and with the help of a free discussion of the abnormal reactions valuable information may be obtained as to previous psychical trauma, home conditions, the patient's personal outlook, and so forth. It is well worth trying in the case of every child patient, although the greater number may give no appreciable result. With adults, however, we often find that there is no necessity for the test. Free discussion with them may be inaugurated from the first without the stepping-stone of Word Association.

The following cases, illustrating results obtained by means of the test, may be of interest.

Louis U. was fourteen when he first came to the Centre, and had been at a Central School for a year. He had a marked stammer ; his manner was truculent and at times decidedly insolent ; he was antagonistic to the treatment from the first, and openly resented any suggestion or criticism in regard to the performance of his exercises. The boy's head master, when we appealed to him, said that this unruly behaviour was completely at variance with his character at school, where he never caused any trouble. The head master's interview with Louis did not result in the slightest improvement, and when, finally, expulsion from the Centre seemed the only course possible, since the boy's behaviour was affecting that of the others, we resorted to the

Word Association Test. We had not tried it sooner because we felt that it could be of little use with so antagonistic a patient, but it solved the difficulty. The significant words were :

Friendly .	Enemy	Falling . .	Hurt
Pride . .	Tears	Sad . . .	Lonely
Sin . .	Punishment	Friend . .	Enemy
Pity . .	Kindness	Fear . . .	Strength

The discussion of these words elicited the following : Louis had been overshadowed, so long as he could remember by his older brother, who had consistently bullied him at home and at his former school, always using his greater physical strength to make the younger boy give in. This brother had been in the habit of taking any of Louis' toys that appealed to him, and had quite recently appropriated a wireless set that Louis had made, for himself. At his former school Louis found, or imagined that he found, boys and masters ' set against him ' by his brother. Since his admission to the Central School, without this older boy, he had for the first time been happy.

It was pointed out to him that something at the Centre must have recalled the conditions at his former school and aroused the antagonism previously mentioned. This explanation he accepted. The result was a complete change of manner on his part and a corresponding improvement in the quality of his work ; he went steadily forward and was cured in a very short time.

He reported progress from time to time after

he had been discharged from the Centre, showing himself more confident and self-assured at each visit. He became head prefect of his school, holding prefects' meetings, making reports at masters' meetings, addressing the school, etc., and any one visiting the Centre when he was present found it difficult to believe that he had ever stammered. This is one of the many instances when the whole personality has been changed for the better by the dispersion of a stammer.

The second case was that of Gerald T., who was admitted when he was twelve years old, having stammered since he was six. At that age he had been sent to stay in Brighton, for reasons of health, with a woman who was not kind to him, and of whom he had been much afraid. Whilst staying there he had stolen five shillings, spent it on sweets, and then lied about it. By the time he returned home the stammer had developed.

His mother lived just outside London, and he spent his holidays with her, living during the term in an orphanage home from which he attended an Elementary School. This home was conducted on highly religious lines which appeared to emphasize unduly the emotional side of the boy's character. He possessed a beautiful singing voice and was in the church choir.

Gerald was highly nervous and very easily discouraged ; he had a distressing inferiority complex, which naturally increased when it was found necessary to send him back to a lower class at school on account of his weakness in arithmetic.

The Word Association Test brought the following

facts to light ᛁ His father had deserted his mother when he was three years old, and they had only met once since. The boy had a strong mother fixation and a corresponding strong sense of antagonism towards his father ; he also brooded over the anomalous position of having a father and yet being in an orphanage.

There was a decided improvement after a discussion of these difficulties, which continued until he left school and, consequently, the Centre. One hopes that he had, by that time, advanced far enough to be able to effect his own ultimate cure.

Dreams.—One has only to read half a dozen authorities on the meaning and interpretation of dreams to realize how easy it is to dogmatize on the subject, and yet how widely divergent are these dogmatic opinions ! They range from simple fortune-telling to the complicated symbolism of Freud and his school, which almost requires a ' dictionary ' for purposes of ' translation '. The whole subject is so wide and—in spite of research—so much *in nubibus*, that we do not feel that any useful purpose would be served by discussing it in a work of this type. Suffice it to say that we consider the dreams of stammerers to be helpful as mental indicators, and that an inquiry into their content should be made in every case.

The effect of the popular cinematograph upon juvenile audiences has recently formed the subject of some considerable controversy. It may be of interest therefore to state that the majority of ' fear ' dreams told us by child stammerers can be traced to the ' pictures '.

Many, too, indicate plainly the patient's inferiority complex, in the Cinderella type of dream. A girl will dream that she is the life and soul of the party, or the best dressed of all present ; a boy that burglars are overpowering his parents and that he ' bashes them all on the head ' and drives them away single-handed. ' I generally dream that I am a wealthy prince riding in a golden chariot ', we were told by a boy of eleven, who also dreamt of ' huge crowds all bowing down to him '.

When a patient has a nightmare that recurs at intervals—be the intervals long or short—it is usually advisable to discuss the content in greater detail. It is interesting to note how often, we might almost say invariably, this discussion disperses the dream. Children especially nearly always report that they ' haven't had that dream since we talked about it '. The suggestion that a dream is dispersed by the telling naturally helps in obtaining such a result.

In conclusion, Nicoll's thesis seems to us to be a reasonable one. He says : ' The incidents of most dreams cover certain episodes, places, and people that are quite familiar. These elements, brought together in an apparently haphazard way in the dream, represent different threads of interest. Each one is, so to speak, a gateway that opens into a big avenue of recollections, feelings, and thoughts.'

Suggestion.—It would be difficult to overrate the importance of suggestion as an essential factor in the cure of stammering—a factor that must underlie all successful treatment. ' The patient having obtained an initial success must be convinced that he is able to repeat it, and so led to perceive that the cure in reality depends on himself,' says Mabel Oswald ; and that 'initial success' is generally quite easy to obtain. Sufficient relaxation can usually be induced on the first day of treatment to cause the stammerer to speak more readily than is customary with him. It can then be pointed out that relaxation has resulted in improvement, however slight, and that deeper ease will mean further progress ; effective treatment has then definitely started. Some patients are, of course, more open to suggestion than others, and these are naturally much easier to help. One boy of ten, for instance, told us that he could speak quite well, but that he could not read aloud although he was very fond of reading to himself ; his statement was tested and found to be painfully true. He was then given an easy poem, and it was suggested that, instead of 'reading' it, he should assimilate a line at a time and then look up and 'say' it. He proceeded to 'say' the entire poem without the slightest hesitation and he was told not to 'read' in future but to adopt this alternative procedure. Naturally this soon became too slow for an intelligent boy, and he was shortly 'reading' more than he was 'saying'. Another child was told to 'think aloud' instead of speaking, with instant success, although it took longer to confirm in his case.

The majority of exercises devised for group work have their greatest value as vehicles for suggestion. The younger the children the more necessary it is to give them definite occupation. But with older children it is possible to explain to a certain extent in simple language that the trouble is psychological, and that the alteration of their habits of thought is a more important part of the treatment than the actual exercises, which are only a means to that end. With adult patients this can be fully discussed, and although breathing and control exercises are necessary at first for all stammerers, these can often be dispensed with in adults long before the defect is definitely cured.

A deplorable amount of faulty suggestion is offered to stammerers. There are, to begin with, the people who constantly iterate the statement that stammering is incurable ; some are broadminded enough to allow that amelioration is possible, others will not even admit so much. To uproot this suggestion from the patient's mind, and to replace it with its opposite, is often a matter of considerable time. A certain number of stammerers are given the impression that because of their disability they are lacking in intelligence. A mother, at the preliminary interview, will say : ' I can't understand it ; my other children are all clever.' One may rest assured that this is not the first time the boy has heard the statement, and its repetition often has the result of making him look stupid because he has for so long thought that he must be.

Another type of suggestion is represented by the case of a boy said to be exactly like his father, who also stammered ; both were much worse, the mother informed us, when the moon was full. And it is hard to believe that any sane person could be guilty of such faulty suggestion as was made in the following case : Fred A. had been attending

7

our Centre for some months, and had made little
progress owing to preoccupation with examination
work; the boy so obviously grudged the time
'wasted' at the Centre that it was finally decided,
with his head master's consent, temporarily to
discharge him. It was understood that he was to
resume attendance so soon as his examination was
over; which he did. Meanwhile a relative had
persuaded the mother to take the boy to a 'specialist', and herself offered to pay the exorbitant
fee demanded by the man she wished them to
consult.

Fred, a very tense and nervous boy, was naturally
strung up for the interview, with the result that
when his breathing was tested his costal movement
was found to be greatly inhibited. According to
the mother, the 'specialist' then told her, *in front*
of the boy, that the lower part of the lungs were in
a semi-paralysed condition, and that if he contracted
pneumonia he was bound to succumb at once, unless
he immediately started breathing exercises. We
give the gentleman the benefit of the doubt since the
mother was naturally extremely agitated when she
came to see us about it; but she is an intelligent
woman, and one not likely to have made a mistake.
It was months before we felt that we had completely
eradicated the fear that had been implanted in
Fred's mind, and had fully convinced him that
muscular rigidity alone was the cause of his costal
tension and spasm.

A stammerer's progress is disconcertingly uneven,
and he is liable to sudden relapses and equally
sudden recoveries. One patient will make great

strides during the first three months of treatment, only to halt for weeks ; another will show no signs of progress for what seems to him an endless time, and then will bound forward as though released from a spring. It is one of our greatest difficulties to make parents understand that a child must not be discouraged during a relapse or when temporarily at a standstill. To tell a sensitive child, who is struggling heroically against odds that are often almost overwhelming him, that he is 'getting no better', or 'will never do any good', is a refinement of cruelty. We admit that there are apparently lazy children who appear to make no effort at improvement, but how often is that 'laziness', a hopeless feeling of *cui bono?* due to the suggestion contained in the thoughtless comments of his parents, and sometimes of his teachers? The stammerer himself is continuously using faulty autosuggestion ; he allows himself to think that he cannot articulate freely certain letters, that he can never speak to particular persons or in given circumstances, etc. We can all remember that sense of sudden inhibition to which we were occasionally liable as, for instance, when we climbed a tree and found that we were unable to descend ; or when our feet were suddenly rooted to the ground because we 'suggested' to ourselves that we could not jump. Stammerers are inhibiting speech every day—some of them do it all day—in exactly the same manner. Is it therefore surprising that the complaint takes a long time to uproot, and that the faulty habit of contra-suggestion persists with such obstinacy in some of the more severe cases ?

A formula of autosuggestion to be used by the patient is of great value, and one of which we make full use. It should hardly be necessary to mention that negative suggestion does more harm than good ; ' I will not stammer ', for instance, generally has the effect of enhancing the trouble. A child of nine informed us when he first came that he had already had ' thought treatment ', which consisted in the formula : ' Every day and in every way my stammer gets better and better.' If ' better ' stood for ' bigger ', the formula was having excellent results ! We find that even Coué's well-known phrase, which we used for several years, may defeat its own ends —with stammerers at any rate—by being too posi- tive. At times it is all too evident to a severe case that he is *not* ' getting better and better ' at the moment. On the other hand, that of Appelt, quoted on page 103 we find admirable, because it is entirely conditional and cannot therefore be gainsaid by the most ' contrary ' mind.

Great care should be exercised by instructors not to give negative or inhibitory advice. Of what use is it to tell one who stammers *not* to think of the letters or words that most embarrass him, or never to be afraid of speaking ? The very orders remind him of his phobia and dread, and help to keep them alive ; and yet methods based on the iteration of such ' rules ' are still all too prevalent.

Suggestion calculated to inculcate habits of mental and physical relaxation not only prevail in estab- lishing those qualities but divert the patient's mind from his former obsession with ' what he is going to say '.

Relaxation.—The basis of all treatment for stammerers—whether individually or in a group—should be relaxation. It is impossible to insist too strongly upon this point ; and it is only necessary to watch the mildest case to see the reason for this insistence. Tension is always present whenever the act of speaking involves a struggle, and this tension must be overcome and replaced by ease before the patient can feel any confidence in his ability to speak. Bluemel, in his latest book, makes light of the necessity for relaxation ; he says that it is 'a minor and not a major factor' in treatment. We cannot but disagree with this view, and with his assertion that children, especially schoolboys, can not and need not learn to relax. He 'tranquillizes' the minds of his patients by means of castanet or clicker signals. The arrangement for some sign to be given to stop the stammerer at the first indication of difficulty is reasonable ; but we cannot agree that the disturbed mind can be 'tranquillized' while awaiting the signal to repeat or to continue what he was going to say. Would not the patient tend, rather, to become tense with anticipatory agitation and anxiety ; a similar agitation, for instance, as is exhibited by the setter setting game ?

With Appelt, on the other hand, we find ourselves in such close agreement that we cannot refrain from quoting at length from his book. He says : ' In order to enable the patient to live up to his autosuggestion, on the one hand, and to counteract the influence of the emotional complex, on the other, it is, according to our experience, to the last extent advisable to cultivate a saturated *feeling* of mental ease. By so doing, the physiological axiom is utilized—namely, when a man practises one and the same feeling over and over again, this feeling will in time dominate the man.

' To this end it is imperative that the patient avoid any too great pressure of volition, and that he speak in the easiest, let us say the most phlegmatic, way possible. Whilst speaking, he must also endeavour to keep up the saturated feeling of ease, and manifest it in the act of speaking itself. . . . The patient should not be afraid of ever being too much at ease. . . . Further, what the patient is going to say should appear to him so indifferent and insignificant in proportion to his endeavour to induce the phlegmatic feeling, that he should be inclined to pay very little attention to the form and construction of his words. The important thing for him is the maintenance of personal ease, and what he is going to say should be of secondary consideration. The patient should work with the greatest determination towards the attainment of ease, of which it is impossible for him to obtain an overplus. . . . The more the patient cultivates the phlegmatic feeling, the more chains of association he forms, which ultimately are able to counteract entirely and to " cover up " the emotional complex. He should take care never to utter a thought unless the feeling of comfort cause it to flow over his lips, as it were ; on no condition should he apply any effort when pronouncing a word ; all his energy, as pointed out before, should be concentrated upon the inducing of the comfortable feeling of ease. The sufferer, in order eventually to be reminded of it automatically, should always keep this thought in mind : " When my feeling of ease is intense enough, the thought *flows* over my lips of itself." This should also form the main theme of his regular autosuggestion.'

This formula of Appelt's we find helpful in practically all cases—even in that of quite young children —except that we use the word " deep " instead of " intense " as being more descriptive of the feeling aimed at.

It can be very difficult for a patient to acquire this ' saturated feeling of mental ease '; he may have to overcome a resistance which to one unused to such cases would seem almost incredible ; and it may take weeks of work in the face of apparent failure before he feels any signs of success. At the Centres, a short time during each session is devoted exclusively to deliberate muscular relaxation, which must of course, be the forerunner of the mental feeling described by Appelt. The children lie on the floor—rugs and cushions being provided for the purpose—and ' think themselves ' into a deeper and deeper feeling of ease. At first the instructor will enumerate the different parts of the muscular system, starting with either the feet or the head, with special insistence on the relaxation of the muscles at the back, shoulders, and neck. Later, the children are able to ' think ' themselves at rest without help. They are told to feel themselves gradually becoming more and more heavy and sleepy, and so soon as they are muscularly relaxed to ' think themselves better ', with the help of their formula of autosuggestion. It is by no means unusual for one

or two children to fall asleep during the short time
—seldom more than ten minutes—allowed for this
relaxation. Needless to say that such results will
not be obtained by the wrong type of instructor,
and that the individual or group under treatment
must co-operate ; it should be superfluous to add
that no one who cannot himself relax can teach
others to do so. A brisk, alert tone or jerky, spasmodic gestures are of no use when ease and repose
are required of the patient. These latter qualities
must be indicated by voice and movement as much
as by the actual words and phrases used, not only
during the period of rest, but for the whole time
that the patient is having treatment. And with
all this it must be the voice of authority—a combination only to be acquired by practice.

Many, when giving instructions on the subject
of relaxation, advocate 'testing' the patient by
some such method as raising an arm or a leg to
ascertain whether he is properly relaxed. We
strongly deprecate this, except as an introductory
aid. If the patient has great difficulty at first, it
may help him to take his hand or arm, gently shake
it to loosen the tension, and let him feel this gradual
ease all over himself. But it is almost impossible
for any one to give himself absolutely to the 'saturated feeling of ease' when he thinks that he may
be 'tested' at any moment. If the patient is
holding himself in readiness for this 'testing', his
relaxation cannot be complete ; and if he is touched,
however lightly, when properly relaxed, it will
cause a considerable jar to his nervous system.
Eric W., a patient of fourteen, who had had a short

period of treatment, supposedly based upon the principles of relaxation, before coming to us, burst out one day with a heartfelt description of his feelings when, so soon as he was beginning to relax comfortably, 'some one started testing him by raising his arm or his leg, and then dropping it.' The boy said that he found it more and more difficult to relax, because he spent the allotted time apprehensively awaiting the 'test'. Incidentally, he was extremely scornful of the command to 'make his mind a blank'—an impossible feat often demanded by those who are not themselves aware of what relaxation means.

Even the practice sometimes put forward of inducing the desired 'feeling of ease' in the patient or patients, by reading 'soothing poems', is unsatisfactory ; it interferes with that complete silence which seems to be productive of the best results. We have always found that the deepest sense of ease is induced by telling the patient to repeat mentally his formula of autosuggestion. The repetition should be slow and drowsy, and it often helps children to tell them to 'feel it sinking into the depths of their minds'.

The sense of ease and well-being that the patient feels as a result of this deliberate relaxation should not be broken when he rises at the finish of the period devoted to this part of the treatment. Anything in the form of a 'signal' to get up should be avoided. The instructor should be careful not to allow his voice to break into the silence ; it should be so low as to form part of the surrounding quiet, and should ensure that the children rise only when they feel ready to move. If this is carried out successfully, the feeling of ease acquired while lying down is continued uninterrupted during the remainder of the session. When the group is co-operating with the instructor this unbroken ease can be effected regardless of numbers, although when it is a question of giving treatment to one patient only it is naturally much more simple. It is by no means uncommon in the latter circumstances for the subject to make not the slightest movement for several minutes after being told that he may rise. Many are so deeply immersed in the feeling of ease as to remain impassive for as long as twenty minutes of conversation following the period of silence.

That hypertonicity is largely responsible for constipation is now being recognized, and we have certainly found that the release of muscular tension has had beneficial results with those stammerers suffering from this condition. The rhythmic movement of the abdominal wall, taught to these patients for the acquiring of diaphragmatic control, would naturally have a share in these results. When Sam V., for example, first came to the Centre his mother was unable to accompany him owing to illness, and we had to wait for more than two months, therefore, before obtaining particulars of his case, during which time he had, of course, worked with the class. When we eventually saw the mother she said that, apart from the stammer, acute constipation had always been Sam's chief trouble, in spite of the endless remedies she had tried. Sam, who was standing by, thereupon remarked that he had been much better in this respect during the last week or two, and his mother agreed that this was so. In this case the improvement could have been in no way due to suggestion, since we had not known of the condition ; it must therefore have been due to the removal of the mental and physical tension to which he had been a victim. Incidentally, he was one of those whose stammer yielded very rapidly to treatment.

A number of schoolboy patients have commented —quite independently of each other—upon their increased prowess in games, and in running and jumping, etc., as a result of losing that inhibitory tension that was impeding them at every turn. And an adult patient, at the end of his second month of treatment, said that his golf had improved to such an extent that his friends were refusing to play with him !

CHAPTER XI

TREATMENT—III

PROPHYLAXIS. — At home, the mother can do much more than is generally realized to prevent stammering at its very inception. Unfortunately, she is more often than not instrumental in fixing the trouble by making too much of the purely physiological stammer with which so many young children begin speech. When a baby is learning to walk he has many a fall before he acquires the co-ordination and control necessary for movement in the desired direction, and at the desired rate of progress. Learning to talk presents the same problem in a much more complicated form. The mechanism used in talking requires infinitely finer and more delicate adjustment than that used in walking.

At the initial stage of speech development the mental process is in advance of the powers of muscular control, and the resulting lack of muscular co-ordination often produces a temporary stammer. If the child is worried and nervous during this period of adjustment he will become conscious of his speech and of the difficulties surrounding its acquisition, and at once the second stage is reached —that of fear or dread of speech—unconscious probably, but none the less potent. Too much attention to the initial difficulties and constant correction or ridicule are usually the cause of this second stage, for which the parents are responsible, either by applying the 'remedy' themselves or by allowing others to do so.

Home Treatment.—Later, when the stammer has become an established fact, many a parent has unintentionally made life harder for the child by mistaken efforts at helping him. The method is the same as that applied by some people to children who are afraid of the dark. They are forced to go along dark passages and into unlighted rooms that they may lose their fear by 'getting used to it'.

On the same principle, the stammering child is made to answer the door or the telephone; he is sent for whenever there are visitors; he has to go out shopping, errands are even invented for him; father or mother is continually calling upon him to read aloud; and in spite of all this 'help' the ungrateful child continues to stammer! One sometimes wonders whether such methods are not even more damaging in their effects than those which prevail in the opposite type of home, where the child meets with anger or blows from impatient parents whose only remedy is to 'shout at him' or to 'scream at him' whenever they hear him in difficulties.

Many a patient has volunteered the information that his stammer is worst when he speaks to his parents, because of his realization of the intense anxiety with which they listen to him. This perception of what parents think they are successfully concealing has been referred to, not only by adult patients but by children so young as twelve. It is of course impossible for parents, with their affection for a child and their sense of responsibility towards him, not to feel anxious and worried over this very trying handicap ; but they should realize how much harder they are making the efforts of the stammerer if they allow him to be aware of their apprehension.   In such a case the sufferer will be acutely conscious that those with whom he associates are over-anxious for him, and he will find reaction to such an atmosphere almost impossible to avoid.

At the opposite extreme is the type of parent that appears to be entirely lacking in sympathetic under-standing—we are not referring to those whose indifference is due to ignorance—and it is heart-rending to realize their unconcern for the suffering which a child can endure as the result of a stammer. They decide to ' do something about it some day ', and meanwhile the child continues to suffer.   One flagrant instance comes to mind, that of Alfred S., the nine-year-old son of a professional man.   We saw the boy three or four times, at intervals of several months, for the purpose of diagnosis and of advising the parents, who were always ' going to arrange ' about treatment.   During one of these visits we were told that Alfred had quite recently had a sudden terrible attack of crying because he ' did so wish he was like other boys '.   This took place three years ago, and still the boy's father has done nothing, although he admitted that after each of the interviews Alfred was better for a time.

Each visit evidently brought renewed hope to the child, only to be followed by bitter disappointment. The reason given for delaying treatment was that Alfred was 'not intelligent enough' to carry out our instructions; and yet his father intended him later to work for one of the most difficult public school scholarships in England !

Again, the mother of a boy of sixteen, herself a highly nervous, efficient individual, told us : ' You have no idea what it is like to live with a stammerer ! Roy often drives me wild with his continual stammering. Of course I try not to let him see that I am impatient.' Such a lack of sympathy has been instrumental in retarding the progress of many cases. It is absurd to suppose that Roy was unaware of this forced restraint on his mother's part ; the fact that he stammered much less when away at school speaks for itself.

Give your stammerer a patient hearing. But it must be a real and not a simulated patience. A stammerer is not only a highly nervous person, but also a very sensitive one, and a pretended patience will be no more helpful to him than open impatience ; he is certain to see through it.

School Treatment.—What of the stammerer at school ? There are, unfortunately, no definite laws for his help and protection ; and yet the time is surely ripe for their formulation. We feel certain that schoolmasters would be the first to welcome definite direction from competent authority. We are faced once again with the lack of uniform opinion on the part of the medical profession, from whom the authoritative statement should come. ' The doctor says that nothing can be done for my boy except the prevention of over-excitement.' 'My doctor says that the child must practise his words until he can say them properly.' And, incredible though it may seem, the mother of one of our cases had been told by a medical man that 'the bad habit *must* be stopped, and that if she could do it by no other means, she was to hit the boy whenever he stammered.'

Most schoolmasters feel an intense sympathy for the stammering child, but have no specialized knowledge of what should be done to help him, and we are continually faced with the victims of their well-meant but mistaken advice, nearly always of the 'trick' variety. George B. (page 80), although an extreme example, is a case in point, and he is only one of many. What, then, can the schoolmaster do to help while the child is undergoing the special course of treatment ?

To begin with, he can definitely forbid stammering.

At first glance such a rule sounds arbitrary and impossible to obey, not to say cruel ; and yet it can be enforced and carried out in a way that will be of real benefit to the stammerer. A little extra trouble is involved certainly—the child will have to write instead of speaking—but is not that extra trouble worth while ? The stammerer should be excused all oral work ; the practice of sending him on messages, or of testing his speech by means of set sentences or reading should be avoided, since it only enhances that 'fear of speech' that underlies all stammering.

The child must of course clearly understand that

silence is imposed to help him, and not because his master has ' no time to wait ' for him ; also that the ban only applies to stammering. Whenever speech flows freely and without effort it should be encouraged. The child will thus have the opportunity for a gradually built up, easy, steady speech which will in time become the rule rather than the exception. James D., after the first week of this régime, informed us enthusiastically that he had never found talking so easy. Having been told that he must not speak unless he found himself able to do so smoothly and effortlessly, and that no one would *expect* him to talk, he immediately felt a release from the strain of anticipatory fear: knowing that he *need* not speak, he was able to do so with an ease which he had never before experienced.

The irony of being able to speak comparatively fluently when it is no longer necessary, or when it is of no importance, is commented upon with feeling by Tompkins. Very few stammerers have difficulty when alone. Many can talk freely to their schoolfellows or to those younger than themselves. When the answer to a question is already known to his listener the patient will have much less difficulty in saying it—often none at all ; but when it is unknown, he is conscious that the information depends upon his ability to impart it, and he is unable to do so. To quote two examples. One boy when asked for his address could not utter a sound ; reference was made by the instructor to his record card, and the moment it was found he gave his address without hesitation. The other was instructed to write the answers to several

8

questions, should he fail in his attempt to do so orally ; he had to write every answer, but so soon as it was written he could speak it fluently. Tompkins instances the case of a man who could say his name only after he had presented his card.

Needless to say that the stammerer is more at his ease with one who is giving him patient and sympathetic attention ; a loud, rough tone, or 'barking' at him, naturally makes him worse, as does any appearance of embarrassment or the 'putting on' of a manner intended to help him. 'I always look the other way when the boy is trying to speak to me,' several schoolmasters have told us. The boy is intensely conscious of this averted look, and he resents it even while he realizes that it is an attempt to make things easier for him.

As the stammer begins to yield to treatment and his self-confidence is returning, there are many ways in which the schoolmaster can assist him to make more rapid progress—as, for instance, putting him in a position of authority in his class, or giving him some definite responsibility. Some of our cases who were patrol leaders in the Scouts said that they never had any difficulty when giving words of command. Many a school prefect has said that he or she never had the slightest trace of hesitation when haranguing or giving orders to juniors ; and one girl of thirteen improved materially in her general speaking after being asked by her head mistress to help in the coaching of three children who were very backward in reading.

General Treatment.—A stammerer often finds that

he can speak more easily to strangers who are not expecting him to stumble, and who will therefore address him normally, than they can to friends and acquaintances who are apt to assume an elaborately unconscious manner when speaking to him. ' I find one of my friends very difficult to talk to ; he is kind and patient, but he watches my lips intently all the time I am speaking.' Charles L., while still attending a treatment Centre, joined a boys' club in which he was a complete stranger ; no one knew that he stammered and no one anticipated it. He found that he was able to speak without a trace of his disability, and the resulting confidence did much to help his ultimate cure.

Tompkins, on the other hand, having suffered cruelly at the hands of strangers, makes a passionate appeal to the general public for more considerate treatment of the stammerer in everyday life. He asks that the policeman, bus-conductor, shop-assistant, telephonist, etc., be given definite instructions in regard to their attitude towards these sufferers, although ' credit is due to a large proportion of public service employees for the sincere " take your time " with which they assist the stammerer ; but generally that comes after the latter has failed to say what he wanted to say, and has been obliged to ask for time.' This is a point upon which we have questioned many patients, and only comparatively few complain of having had inconsiderate treatment ; the majority say that people are generally kind and patient. Most of our schoolboy cases relate that their contemporaries are sympathetic, and often that they try to be helpful ; surprisingly few meet with derision and mockery, and in nearly every instance such an attitude is severely reprimanded so soon as the master is aware of it. Schoolfellows too have often encouraged our patients by commenting upon their improved speech when parents and teachers have not thought to remark upon it.

The adult has, as a rule, more to encounter than the child at school ; he has to buy his own ticket, order his own meals in a restaurant, and must himself ask the way of the policeman or the casual passer-by. There are times of course when the stammerer is treated with what almost amounts to deliberate cruelty by impatient persons, or by those utterly lacking in imagination. Such occurrences are comparatively rare, but they ought to be impossible.

One of our patient's commented with great indignation upon a ' talkie ' she had recently witnessed, in which one of the characters was a stammerer. She said that half the audience found no humour in the situation, but that the remainder laughed heartily. Another patient, a born comedian, who never stammered when acting, told us of having been given the part of a stammerer in a school play. Every one was delighted with his performance. ' The audience—fellow-scholars and their relations —roared with laughter whenever he stammered ! '

A stammering character is very seldom seen on the stage, but the fact that such a performance is calculated to attract an audience seems to us to be an unhappy state of affairs. There is nothing humorous in such an affliction as stammering ; nor

are the unintelligible sounds made by one with a
cleft palate comic, and yet several years ago an
actor in a London theatre convulsed his audience
with an imitation of such ' speech '. Is not this
rather a reflection upon our present-day civilization
with its boasted knowledge of psychology ? Public
opinion should surely bar performances calculated
to ridicule personal infirmities.

Age for Treatment.—At first it was thought that
the best results would be obtained at treatment
Centres by admitting the children at an early age,
that is to say, at seven, or even younger. It was
considered advisable to give treatment before the
habit had had time to become definitely fixed.
Experience, however, has shown that these younger
children require a longer time for treatment, and
that there is, with them, a greater tendency to
relapse. They are not, as a rule, sufficiently independent or self-reliant ; they are apt to rely entirely
upon the help given them at the Centre, and although
they often progress admirably while actually attending, relapse so soon as they are required to depend
upon themselves. A little girl of six, for example,
progressed so favourably as to be discharged at
the end of one term, only to need readmission six
months later.

If it were possible to have these younger children
under daily supervision the results would certainly
be much more satisfactory. But visiting the Centre
twice a week only, and being left to carry out
instructions by themselves between these visits,
a child cannot in general be pronounced definitely
cured until a very long time has elapsed. Often,

too, he will tend to grow tired of this lengthy
process ; he may become careless and inattentive
in the class, and cease all home practising. In
such cases there is usually a relapse which adds
yet further to the child's discouragement.

Not that one would wish to imply that it is of no
use to give treatment to younger children—many
of these benefit greatly ; but if a child under eight
is to make any appreciable progress he must have
constant help, and with the Elementary School
children who attend our Centres this is not an easy
matter. Both mother and teacher have, as a rule,
too much to do to be able to spare time for the
help and attention they would wish to give ; and
only an older child can follow instructions system-
atically by himself.

The treatment of a very young child is best
carried out with the assistance of his mother or
nurse. She accompanies him on his visits, helps
him to carry out the instructions at home, reports
progress, and generally aids and encourages him.
By the time he is nine years old, unless he is of the
very irresponsible type, he can begin to take himself
in hand ; supervision is still necessary at this stage,
but should be unobtrusive ; the patient's confidence
in himself, and his consequent progress, are greatly
assisted if he feels independent and self-reliant.
When he reaches the age of twelve or so he has
developed a certain sense of responsibility, his
powers of concentration are greater, he is beginning
to realize what a handicap in life his stammer would
prove if it persisted. His determination to carry
out what he has undertaken upholds him through

obstacles and temporary relapses that frequently defeat his junior.

Many authorities maintain that the cure of stammering becomes increasingly difficult as the patient grows older, and that by the time he is grown up it has become impossible to do more than alleviate the trouble. This view is one that we cannot admit; in our experience the adult stammerer has often been the more rapidly cured. We agree with Chervin that 'Age is never an obstacle to success so long as determination and courage are not lacking.' Since treatment depends upon the patient's understanding and willing co-operation, the adult is, as a rule, the more rapidly cured. A child, when answering questions and giving an account of himself, is not only held back, by shyness and self-consciousness—a dislike of 'giving himself away'—he is further impeded by the lack of a suitable vocabulary with which to express himself. Any discussions regarding conflicts, repressions, and difficulties generally is much easier with the adult patient, who will, in addition, be able to give a more detailed and comprehensive history. Further, the adult comes for treatment with a more definite incentive, more sense of responsibility, and a greater determination to do all that is needful to effect his cure, all this counteracting the fact that the stammer has probably taken deeper roots with the passing years.

Class Treatment.—Every patient is an individual case, requiring individual attention, but that does not mean that working in a group is ineffective. Admittedly, no two in a class will stammer alike, but they will have a number of traits in common, such as nervous and muscular tension, fear of speech, a greater or lesser sense of inferiority, and so forth. The alleviation of these difficulties is helped rather than hindered by the presence of fellow-sufferers. Parents are often anxious at first lest a mild stammer become worse by mixing with more severe cases, but experience has shown this anxiety to be unfounded. There is sometimes a temporary increase of stammering when a patient first begins treatment, whether alone or in a class, because so often he will try to do too much, and between over-eagerness and the inability to relax the trouble may be intensified for a few days. But when parents have complained of a relapse after favourable progress had been made, we invariably find that this is due to some other cause, and not, as they think, to imitation of a more acute stammer.

When a child first comes to a Centre his reaction to the class is more often than not one of relief. Hitherto, unless he has known a number of other stammerers, he has had a sense of isolation, he has felt himself to be an outcast and in some way blameworthy, he has wondered bitterly why he alone should be different from the rest of mankind. All this is changed when he finds himself surrounded by fellow-sufferers ; as his work with the class advances he will find further encouragement in noticing that his trouble is not so marked as that of A ; that improvement is being made by B and C, which he can emulate ; that D and E have practically stopped stammering and are on the point of being discharged, thus proving the possibility of a cure in his own case.

Again, the intensely nervous child, or one that is painfully shy, can be allowed to fade into the background at first, should he feel so inclined, and remain in comfortable obscurity until he feels more sure of himself. Among younger children this apparent neglect is often very helpful ; we have had several whose inhibitory shyness has made them almost incapable of joining in with the rest of the class until they have become accustomed to their new surroundings. We retain vivid recollections of one such case, a little boy of eight—a thin, depressed, miserable-looking child who wept copiously at being left by his mother, and who moped through the allotted time without attempting to work with the others. A few days later the children were finishing the session with acting, and the instructor asked for some one to take the part of a policeman ; Billy volunteered and gave an admirable performance, entering into the game with spirit and thoroughly enjoying himself. His histrionic success removed the barrier of shyness, and with it his refusal to co-operate with the other members of the class.

When a child is having private treatment he is bound to be the centre of attention, and the shy child derives little benefit at first, owing to his self-consciousness. The spirit of emulation too is absent, and there is nothing to prevent that feeling of isolation and of ' difference ' which all stammerers carry about with them. We find therefore that with younger children the advantages of class treatment more than compensate for the disadvantages. It is certainly not easy to find time and opportunity for the individual work necessary in every case, especially if the instructor is single-handed ; but with careful arrangement this can be done, and by so doing the only serious drawback to class treatment for stammering children is removed.

When a patient is working alone the method will depend entirely upon his personal needs, but when a number are to be given treatment in a group the instructor must arrange exercises, etc., that will benefit the class as a whole. The basic factors of suggestion, relaxation, and rhythmic co-ordination must always be the foundations of treatment ; but so much depends upon the personality of the instructor and the individual requirements of members of the group that no hard and fast rules can be laid down for the application of these principles.

We will endeavour to give a rough outline of a class of children at work, but the details must inevitably depend upon the circumstances already mentioned.

In the first place, the children must acquire as much ease as possible in order to derive the utmost benefit from their various exercises. Sitting at his desk, each child should allow the ' feeling of ease ' to spread through his whole body and gradually invade his mind. He does not find the mental ease difficult when once he has acquired muscular relaxation ; nor is there fear of speech in a class where every one is a stammerer, anticipatory dread is therefore eliminated.

Breathing exercises follow ; smooth, rhythmic movement is essential ; there must be no effort and no strain. Frequent pauses should be made so as to prevent any possibility of muscular tension, each pause being a reminder to the child of the importance of maintaining ease throughout.

Next, rhythmic movements of the abdominal wall are practised, and when flexibility has been attained these movements are combined with the breathing in order to obtain control of the respiratory action. Explanations suited to the age of the patients may be given from time to time in order to keep alive their interest in the exercises.

After this the children lie on the floor for the complete relaxation to which reference has already been made on page 103.

When they have returned to their places they may read, recite, act, play some form of speech game, or practice rhythmic movement ; mime gestures are a great help in restoring muscular co-ordination. Alternatively, movement may occasionally take the place of the breathing and control exercises in order to vary the routine.

The children themselves must clearly understand that whatever they are asked to do during the last part of the session is not to be regarded as a speech test, but as a test of their powers of relaxation. ' When my feeling of ease is deep enough the thought flows over my lips of itself.' If a child stammers it shows that his ' ease ' is not deep enough ; let him therefore relax further, rather than ' try to say it again '. Nor must the child be constantly reminded of his breathing and control processes ; these should—through relaxation and the effect of rhythmic exercises—adjust themselves. We frankly admit having been guilty of error in this respect in the past ; of having told our patients always to ' breathe before speaking ', and to ' control ' consciously during speech ; but we now realize that this is definitely wrong.   As we have said before, speech and its attendant processes should be automatic, and a stammerer's attention should be drawn away from, and not towards, the muscular movements involved.

To make these points quite clear let us imagine an instructor testing the speech of a patient who has been attending a Centre for three or four months— a severe case, but one that is showing signs of improvement.   The child can relax muscularly when he is concentrating on that alone, but still has great difficulty in doing so while speaking.   The instructor has asked him to repeat one verse of any poem that he has been learning lately.

The patient makes an effort to begin, tension and spasm interfere, and he is speechless.

(*Old Style*)

Instructor: 'Let yourself relax. Now quietly breathe in and say the first line slowly, drawing in your " control muscle " while you are speaking ' (diaphragmatic control).

(*New Style*)

Relax and wait until your feeling of ease is deep enough.   Take your time.

Patient : Endeavours to follow these instructions, but probably takes in far more breath than he needs, and muscular rigidity and spasm return.

Endeavours to do so, but stiffens as soon as he tries to articulate.

(Old Style)
Instructor : Gives the same orders as before.

(New Style)
'Think of nothing but " ease " ; let your muscles become heavier and heavier. There is no need to worry over what you are going to say, as you already know it by heart; you can therefore give the whole of your mind to thinking of ease.'

Patient : Breathes, succeeds in forcing out the first three or four words, but can do no more.

Succeeds in saying three or four words fluently, but cannot prevent tension from supervening.

Instructor : Repeats the order to breathe and control with slightly varied wording. This continues until the patient has struggled through the verse— the instructor being under the impression that, having once started, the child must finish somehow, in order to prevent a false sense of failure.

Stops him at first sign of difficulty. 'That was splendid. You said half a line quite smoothly, and that is infinitely better than a whole poem stammered. Let us now see whether ease will carry you a little farther. If it won't, never mind ; you will be relaxing more easily next time you come here, and you can say it then.'

It will be seen at a glance how much more encouraging to the child is the second method.

When planning the form which the oral test of 'ease' is to take, the instructor must bear in mind the special needs of every member of the group. It is, for instance, advisable when a new-comer with a severe stammer is first admitted to allow no individual speaking or reading aloud until he has mastered the rudiments of relaxation. Or, again, if one or two members of the class show signs of extreme muscular inco-ordination, the instructor can arrange for the whole group to practise mime and other rhythmic movements for several successive sessions. A capable instructor will, in fact, be continually devising new angles of approach to the various exercises, in order to keep alive the children's interest in the task of curing themselves.

It will be seen from the foregoing paragraphs how impossible it is to dogmatize about the details of group management, or to set down tables of exercises for treatment that must always be adapted to the temperamental requirements of the class as a whole. One can therefore give no more than the merest indication of class treatment ; experience alone can teach the instructor how to fill in the details.

Discipline.—The question of discipline in these classes sometimes presents difficulty. The fact that stammerers are nervous persons who must be treated with special consideration and must not be unduly rebuked has been known to result in the complete abandonment of discipline, and one has seen a group of only four children in a constant uproar because they ' must not be thwarted ', or have their nervous system upset by severity.

Harsh methods and undue restraint are naturally bad for the nervous system of any child ; but lack of all restraint and continual noise are equally bad. The stammerer needs mental and physical quiet above all things, and these can only be achieved in an atmosphere of calm and repose. So soon as the patient learns what is meant by ease and relaxation he becomes interested in the comfort and security obtained thereby, and is anxious to continue farther on the same lines. The majority of stammerers definitely welcome discipline and order ; even the most difficult cases do so subconsciously.

Discipline is of course harder to obtain among younger children, but even with these it can be done ; and in this discipline through relaxation the personality of the instructor counts more than in anything else. Voice and gesture must be quiet and suggestive of repose. A raised voice or jerky utterance is of no use when instructing those whose need is a rhythmic and restful background for all that they do. If, however, the children are concerned with their own progress, and anxious to do the best they can to ensure a lasting cure, the question of discipline hardly arises. The majority are keenly interested, especially if it is made clear to them from the start that progress depends entirely upon themselves, and that no one but the stammerer can effect his cure.

Incentive.—We feel that one reason for the slower progress made by younger children may be the lack of a definite incentive, without which they soon lose heart and become troublesome and inattentive. Many, however, will respond readily to the suggestion of trying to effect a cure by a given date—next birthday, for instance, or the beginning of a new year. Older children are determined to be cured by the time they leave school. We have had many cases of boys and girls who, having won scholarships, wished to make a new start at the Central or Secondary School. The nature of the incentive varies with each case, and progress is always more rapid when the patient is working towards a specific goal. The incentive in a certain number of cases is the wish to undertake some form of public speaking; an ambition that has hitherto been regarded as hopeless, not to say ludicrous. The knowledge that such a career will be within the bounds of possibility when the stammer has been overcome is a great encouragement to progress.

The father of one of our schoolboy patients, thinking that his son was not improving as quickly as he might, promised the boy a shilling for every day without a stammer during his holidays; the results were excellent, if somewhat expensive!

CHAPTER XII

CONCLUSION

IN conclusion we feel that in this brief survey of the nature and treatment of stammering we have by no means exhausted the subject ; but we hope to have paved the way for further investigation.

The book is based on the personal experience of ten years of research and its practical application. Every year we find it necessary to emphasize more strongly the paramount importance of a complete investigation of each case from every point of view—physical, psychological, and environmental. Often the discovery of some apparently trivial detail will alter the whole aspect of a case.

Equally important is the application of the principles of mental and physical relaxation in treatment.

Every stammerer is an individual case, but this in no way contradicts our statement that class treatment is the best method for dealing with young children.

It is our earnest wish that the perusal of these pages may result in a message of hope to the stammerer, some enlightenment to his parents and teachers, and a more reasonable attitude on the part of the general public towards those oppressed with this distressing affliction.

BIBLIOGRAPHY

ADLER : *Individual Psychology.* 1924.

APPELT : *Stammering and Its Permanent Cure.* 1911.

BLUEMEL : *Stammering and Cognate Defects of Speech.*

CAMERON : *The Nervous Child.* 1929.

CORIAT : *Stammering, a Psychoanalytical Interpretation.* 1928.

CULPIN : *The Nervous Patient.* 1924.

GILLESPIE : ' Psychology and Psychopathology of Childhood ', *Brit. Med. Jour.*, Nov. 15th, 1930.

KERR : *Fundamentals of School Health.* 1926.

McCORMAC : *Cause and Cure of Hesitation of Speech or Stammering.* 1828.

TOMPKINS : ' Stammering Not an Amnesia ', *New York Med. Jour.*, Nov. 1st, 1919, etc.

INDEX

For Product Safety Concerns and Information please contact our EU
representative GPSR@taylorandfrancis.com
Taylor & Francis Verlag GmbH, Kaufingerstraße 24, 80331 München, Germany